Family Therapy & Chronic Illness

Family Therapy & Chronic Illness

JOAN D. ATWOOD & CONCETTA GALLO
(and Contributors)

ALDINETRANSACTION
A Division of Transaction Publishers
New Brunswick (U.S.A.) and London (U.K.)

Library of Congress Catalog Number: 2009036625
ISBN: 978-0-202-36335-6
Printed in the United States of America

Library of Congress Cataloging-in-Publication Data

Family therapy and chronic illness / [edited by] Joan D. Atwood, Concetta Gallo, and contributors.
     p. cm.
Includes bibliographical references and index.
ISBN 978-0-202-36335-6
    1. Family psychotherapy. 2. Mental illness--Treatment. 3. Chronically ill--Treatment. I. Atwood, Joan D. II. Gallo, Concetta.

RC488.5.F33415 2009
616.89'156--dc22

                  2009036625

For My Children

who continually amaze me with their intelligence,
competence and kindness:

Debra Gibbons

Barbara Winnik

Lisa Gaudioso

Janine Collier

Brian Atwood

I love you all, MaMa

(JDA)

With all my love and gratitude to the Gallo family from 78th Street, and to my brother, Peter: We, two, are left and I want you to know that I cherish you and the memories we can make and continue to share.

(CG)

Dedication

This book is dedicated to my daughter, Barbara, who passed away from lung cancer last year. I will be forever thankful that I was blessed with a daughter whose kindness, courage, and compassion taught me the greatest lesson in my life. Your spirit, love, and energy live on in all of us. We will love you forever, Babsie.

JDA

This book is dedicated to the memory of my sister, Maria, with whom I learned, shared, and created family stories. Thank you for showing me the true meaning of courage as you fought the most difficult battle of your life. Your life, your memory, and your love will serve as daily reminders for me. Mary, the greatest privilege of my life was to be your baby sister.

Forever, Cetta

Contents

Introduction

Recently, there has been an increased recognition of the importance of collaboration between the family medical and family therapy fields. In many cases, family therapists and family physicians are part of the same treatment team. However, this innovative treatment approach is still relatively rare and much more collaboration is needed. It is the purpose of this book to familiarize family therapists with some of the effects of chronic illnesses on family members. It is also our hope that family physicians may come to recognize some of the issues and problems that couples and families with a chronically-ill member may experience, and the importance of a family therapist as part of the team.

Approximately, 33.1 million people have some degree of limited activity due to chronic illness. For the purposes of this text, an illness is considered to be chronic if it is a persistent, progressive, and degenerative disease. Since the publication of *Family Systems Medicine* in 1982, there has been an increased recognition of the importance of addressing the therapy needs of medical patients and their families within the context of a biopsychosocial model. While research studies have focused on such chronic illnesses as diabetes, heart disease, and cancer and their effect on the individual; the couple and other family members' therapy needs have not received comparable attention. There is a need for more systemically-oriented therapy research to address the complex needs of couples and families coping with chronic illness.

It is the purpose of this book to address some of the issues and problems that couples and families with a chronically-ill member may experience. Implications for conducting therapy with a chronically ill client and his/her family are considered throughout the book.

Chronic illness is not simply an individual subjective experience; it has biological, interpersonal, and social factors. The definition or meaning an individual gives to an illness is profoundly influenced by and influences that person's social world. The social culture and the social networks shape and are shaped by the individual's experiences. The meaning of the illness is shared and negotiated in everyday interactions and it is deeply embedded in the social world. As such it is inseparable from the structure and processes that constitute that social world. To explore the definitional processes involved in chronic illness is to explore the individual's interpersonal relationships and the resultant meaning system.

Unexpected, health-related life events raise many questions for therapists and other health service providers. What are the factors that determine the onset of serious, chronic, and degenerative diseases and how does the progression of an illness affect families? To what extent does gender, the life cycle stage of the players at the onset of the illness (childhood/adulthood), roles, couple relationships, social support systems, and finances contribute to the way families cope? Can family systems be strengthened rather than weakened in the face of health problems? How do marital and family dynamics, belief systems, rules, and boundaries determine the physical well-being of its members and their ability to adapt to physical health problems? This book provides a foundation for understanding the role a chronic illness plays in family systems and the implications for effective intervention. Case material will illustrate this point.

A husband and wife walk into a therapist's office; the wife's primary care physician has referred them to the therapist. The presenting problem is depression due to the wife's recent diagnosis of multiple sclerosis (MS). This is coupled with the fact that the youngest of the couple's four children left home a few months earlier for college. The wife's physician and therapist both believe themselves to be post-modern and wholistic in their approach. The progression of the wife's MS has left her unable to walk without a wheelchair and to stand. However, the home the couple lives in has not been modified to accommodate the wife's changing physical condition. Each weekend morning the husband asks his wife if she has made the coffee. Each weekend morning the wife must "confess" that she has not and both feel badly. The husband interprets her not making the coffee as something she has willfully chosen not to do, one of the few things he requests of her since her diagnosis. She feels more inadequate and that she has failed him. The therapist notes that the coffeepot cannot be reached from her wheelchair.

Both husband and wife can remember the time, not so long ago when she made him coffee not just on the weekends but on the weekdays as well. Every morning she got up and prepared the coffee, as he got ready for work. Like so many couples of their age group, their marriage was a "traditional" one. He got up and went to work and she stayed home and took care of their children, their home, and him. He has been a good and faithful husband, he went to work everyday, then came home to dinner. On the weekends he mowed the lawn and painted the garage door. She stayed home and cooked the meals, cleaned the house, took care of the children, and planned the family's weekend visits, holidays, and other social activities.

Now since her diagnosis both of them have had to deal with a change in their established roles. Now after work he must do the laundry, wash the dinner dishes, and tend to some other household chores. On the weekends, he must still mow the lawn and paint the garage but now he must also go to the supermarket, vacuum the rugs, and wash the kitchen floor. Is it too much to ask that twice a week he get up to a fresh pot of coffee that was made for him? Is it too much to ask that twice a week, she make him the coffee? He does not think it is too much to ask.

Not only is the wife suffering from MS and grieving the loss of daily activity, but she is also grieving the loss of her identity as the homemaker and as his wife. She watches as he leaves each morning without a warm cup of coffee that she once dutifully made for him. She watches as he comes home from work and eats the much more simple dinner she has prepared or on the evening when she is especially tired, as they both share the fast food he has picked up on the way home. She watches as he washes the dishes and then goes into the basement to do a load of laundry. She must take solace in the fact that she is still able to sit on the couch and fold the laundry, which he has washed and dried. She also asks herself, is it too much for him to expect her to make him a cup of coffee twice a week? And she too knows the answer that it is not. She feels even worse, she knows that she has disappointed him and she slips hopelessly into a deeper and deeper depression.

Both husband and wife must deal with her MS but they must also deal with their changed roles and the impact it has had on their marriage and on their definitions of them selves. These definitions are socially established, in fact were socially established for them. These definitions have been taught to them by their families, by their society, and they have internalized them. These definitions have been socially constructed and the therapist working with this couple requires systemic skills, and a minimum knowledge of the symptoms of MS, but additionally must also have an understanding of the social roles of the couple and how these roles have come to define them-selves as who they are not only to each other but also to themselves.

Literature dealing with chronic illness on a biopsychosocial level, only pays lip service to the "social aspect." The expectation that she as the woman makes the coffee is rooted in the language that she must "confess" that she has not. One confesses to a crime, not to not making a cup of coffee. If it was he who had been diagnosed with MS, a confrontation to the problem may not mean changing the physical layout of the home even if it meant that she went to work. Would the couple be discussing that now that she is working, she is upset that on the weekends he does not make her coffee? No, because both the couple and the therapist buy into the social construction of reality, that it is the woman who does such chores as make the coffee. Perhaps, the couple would have to deal with other problems such as his feeling incompetent because he cannot economically provide for his family.

If one wants to look at chronic illness from a "biopsychosocial" aspect than one must also explore the sociological implications on the diagnosis to the individual's sense of self and identity. When an individual becomes chronically ill, the individual must not only deal with the physical and or physiological component of the illness, but the illness affects the person psychologically, spiritually, and sociologically as well.

There is a scarcity of literature on families with a chronically ill member experiencing the feelings of anomie, for example. The feelings of normlessness that having a chronic illness can cause. The feeling of not knowing what is expected of you. Society tells us what is expected of us as adults and most of us conform to this expectation. But being diagnosed with a chronic illness can lead both the individual and his/her family into a feeling of normlessness, the social expectations have changed and they do not understand their own selves, their own identities, let alone their roles. Their taken for granted reality has changed sometimes overnight or in a simple visit to a doctor's office.

This book approaches chronic illness from a leading edge perspective. The chapters move between analytical narrative therapy based in a social constructionist framework into a more "hands on" approach illustrating the concepts with case material. This approach enables therapists to listen very expertly and attentively to extraordinarily complicated narratives. These narratives are told in words, gestures, silences, tracings, images, and physical findings. These narratives or stories are then integrated into a coherent whole. The therapist is the interpreter of these often contra-dictory accounts of events that are, by definition, difficult to tell: pain, suffering, worry, anguish, the sense of something just not being right. These stories, feelings and emotions are very difficult to describe in words so the clients have very demanding "telling" tasks while therapists have very demanding "listening" tasks. As previously noted, being diagnosed with a chronic illness can change every aspect of a person's life. This book will undertake the task of doing family therapy from a post-modern social constructionist origin with a family in which one or more of its members have been diagnosed with a chronic illness.

For example, in discussing such diseases as breast cancer it is important to realize that the diagnosis of such a disease to a female patient can have an impact on the woman's sense of self and her identity. The mastectomy can cause a change in her identity and her sense of self. These terms are distinct in sociological theory especially in symbolic interactionist theory where identity is located as an aspect of self. However, both self and identity are socially constructed. The self is an ever-evolving process that is socially constructed. I am to myself what society says that I am. The self is a social object that the actor acts towards. An individual comes to see self in interactions with others. One's self is pointed out and defined socially. The individual becomes an object to herself because of others. As a woman, part of her self is, according to society, her body, her physical shape including her breasts. There is no doubt that breasts play an enormous part in a woman's definition of her self and in her identity. Losing a breast can alter the woman's view of herself as an object because of society's definition of what a woman is. This can impact on her relationship with her husband and her family. She may see herself as she believes her husband is seeing her (less than a woman) and may internalize his imagined reaction into her identity. In working with this couple, it is important to realize that even though the husband may reassure her that she is just as beautiful and desirable to him, she may in viewing herself as a social object, not believe him.

One's identity is who one tells the self one is and what one announces to others that one is. A woman's identity has also been changed as she gets labeled as someone with breast cancer or someone who has had a mastectomy. This label will impact on her identity and thus on her self and on her relationships with others, especially her primary group, her family. Likewise, the husband may also be internalizing society's definition of a woman.

If we return, to the example we started with we can see that the wife's inability to make her husband coffee may impact on her self as a woman and her identity as a wife. Her change in self will mean a change in all the system's parts and will mark a change in the husband's identity. The therapist must be aware of this as he/she deals with the couple.

In reading the chapters of this book, it is important for the reader to realize that he/she is not embarking on territory that has not been previously explored but on a trip, which entails looking at the same terrain from a different approach.

This book is more than an introduction to chronic illness issues. It focuses on the most current theoretical issues in the field written by the top experts in the field. Each chapter has its own bibliography with suggestions for further reading.

The field of family therapy is comparatively new. There is no doubt that it has borrowed from a number of other disciplines including both the natural and social sciences. One aspect of family therapy that has been especially intriguing to the editors is its eclectic approach. In essence, there is no one right way to do therapy. There are different schools of thought on therapeutic theories, approaches, and interventions. This book hopes to present to its readers an eclectic approach to chronic illness and the family. To this end, the editors invited authors from a variety of fields to write about the changing family, specific chronic illnesses, family stories, narratives, and treatment. It is the unique aspect of the collection of these chapters that the editors hope will be the lasting contribution to the field of family therapy. Below is a brief synopsis of each chapter. It is the hope of the editors that these will entice the reader.

Chapter One explores the relationship between chronic illness sympathology, and the roles of family members. Specifically, the chapter contends that the roles of family members develop in response to living with a family member who has a chronic illness, and are learned through family stories. Emphasis is given to the interrelationship of the role and behavior of the chronically-ill member, and the role and behavior of the caregiver. Additionally, the sociological theory of alternation will be briefly discussed as a prelude to an in-depth discussion of Narrative Family Therapy theory. This will then lead into a discussion of family stories and narratives. Finally, a case study of James and Connie Bellasera (pseudonyms) will be used to emphasize the importance of family stories on the roles family members embrace, and to exemplify the application of White's Narrative Family Therapy.

It is the purpose of Chapter Two to address some of the issues and problems that couples and families with a chronically-ill member may experience, taking life cycle issues into consideration. A distinction is made between the illness experience and the illness behavior. To this, the authors have added the illness meaning: the social and psychological definitions given to the illness and the resultant scripts taken on by the ill member, the couple, and other family members. Implications for therapy are considered throughout the chapter.

Chapter Three provides readers with an understanding of how cultural factors play a significant role within families who have members with chronic illness, disability, and secondary disabling conditions. The significance of how cultural factors will contribute to the coping, adjusting, caring and managing of family members who acquired chronic illnesses and secondary disabling conditions will be presented and discussed in detail. A summary and recommendations of cultural competence skills for working with families from diverse cultural and ethnic backgrounds will be presented. The challenge of a paradigm shift that has taken place and for future family therapy or counseling applications in a culturally diverse American society are discussed and hopefully, this compilation of well researched information will enhance your studies and research, and your professional ethics practice in this rewarding profession.

Chapter Four hopes that a greater understanding of the social nature of marriage and family life will come by examining the changes of U.S. families in recent decades, the topic addressed by sociologists Doyle McCarthy and Sondra Farganis in "The Changing American Family." The authors describe a climate of change in people's perceptions of themselves, their workaday lives, and in marriage and family life—changes occurring in the last half century. Most importantly, they report evidence for a shift from a relatively dominant standard of family life: *"the family" (the cultural and "traditional" ideal) has been replaced by an acceptance of more varied institutional forms—"families" or "diversity" in families.* These findings represent changes in both collective behavior and public opinion: *in people's behaviors* (with respect to marrying, divorcing, remarrying, parenting), *in the increasingly diverse types of households* (one- or two-parent households, same-sex or opposite-sex parents, natural and adoptive parents, families with children and stepchildren), and changes *in the ways people think about and evaluate the institutions of marriage and family*—changes in the cultures people draw from and use in their own lives and how they evaluate others' lives. McCarthy and Farganis conclude their chapter with proposals for a public family sociology—a sociology accessible to an educated lay public and to family practitioners and therapists.

Chapter Five explores the family experience of Multiple Sclerosis (MS). Recently, there has been an increased recognition of the importance of addressing the counseling needs of MS couples and their families, signaling the need for couple-oriented approaches to address the complex needs of couples coping with MS. Multiple sclerosis is a chronic, progressive, and degenerative neurological disease that produces a breakdown of the myelin sheath that surrounds central nervous system axons. It is the purpose of this chapter to address some of the issues and problems MS couples may experience, taking life cycle issues into consideration. A distinction is made between the illness *experience* and the illness *behavior*. To this is added the illness *meaning*, the social and psychological definitions given to the illness and the resultant scripts taken on by the couple and by family members. A four stage therapeutic model based on social constructionist assumptions is then presented and illustrated by case material.

Chapter Six discusses the definition of Irritable Bowel Syndrome (IBS), its impact on individuals, couples, and families taking into consideration cultural factors, economic factors, life cycle issues, and traditional medical models. Deficit assumptions surrounding therapy with the chronically ill, including the psyshosomatic model, standardized family assessments, family of origin issues, object relations, and solution-focused models of therapy are explored.

Chapter Seven on mindfulness-based family therapy by Dr. Anthony R. Quintiliani, is an attempt to expand the use of mindfulness-based interventions in family therapy practice. The chapter serves as a partial remedy to the relative dearth of mindfulness-based interventions in family therapy for chronic conditions. Specific details on clinical applications of various mindfulness-based interventions have been noted to allow replication by family therapists.

Chapter Eight explores the social construction of the caregiver self, reviews common interventions to improve caregiver health, discusses the potential value of therapeutic techniques grounded in social constructionist theory, and argues that family physicians serve as a critical gateway to mental health care for at-risk caregivers. Caring for aging, chronically-ill parents is becoming a way of life for many Americans. The socially constructed "caregiver self" can incorporate positive elements from the previous self-identity, or it can overwhelm the previous self-identity putting the caregiver at great risk for psychological and physiological crisis. How the caregiver experiences their role transformation, how well they accept and manage the integration of their past self and their new self, and how they perceive their social world to experience their new role, will determine the caregiver self-identity and the ability of the caregiver to provide quality care while maintaining a high quality life of their own.

Chapter Nine, entitled "A Good Death" is aimed at describing symptom management strategies medical professionals have used in responding to and preventing requests of terminally-ill patients for assisted dying. The study involves analysis of written stories from critical care professionals who agreed to describe their experiences with a request for assisted dying. Critical care professionals discussed their refusal to support such patient requests and described their attempts to control the circumstances of dying by controlling symptoms, all the while taking into consideration the patient's and family wishes. Professionals who denied ever receiving requests for assisted death described preventative symptom management. Two themes emerged from the participant's stories: alternative strategies for assisted death and prevention of requests for assisted death. The participants shared many examples of clinical interventions and other responses to relieve or prevent suffering including physical, emotional, and spiritual care practices; comfort and medication management; and service as teacher-advocate. All of the respondents who had received requests for assisted death and those who had not used a variety of similar symptom management approaches to alleviate suffering. In doing so, they upheld current standards of both their professional and specialty organizations.

1

The Stories of Chronic Illness: Narrative Roles and Family Therapy

Concetta Gallo

Abstract

The purpose of this chapter is to explore chronic illness from a perspective of learned helplessness. This was learned through family stories. Varying roles in the family system will be examined. Specifically, the role and behavior of the chronically-ill member and the role of the caregiver will be discussed. The sociological theory of alternation will be briefly discussed as a prelude to an in-depth discussion of Narrative Family Therapy theory. This will lead into a discussion of family stories and narratives. Finally, a case study of James and Connie Bellasera will be used to emphasize the importance of family stories on the roles members embrace, and to exemplify the application of White's Narrative Family Therapy.

Chronic illness and family therapy are often discussed within the context of conducting therapy with chronically-ill patients and their families. The onset of a chronic illness can cause chaos in an otherwise well-functioning family. The impact of a chronic illness on a dysfunctional family will be more severe.

Similarly, the idea of family stories in family therapy is within the context of stories within the therapy sessions. There is however, a scarcity of literature on how family stories, family roles, and chronic illnesses are interrelated. From this perspective, we may ask, can members of a family system adapt certain roles in response to a family member being diagnosed with a chronic illness? Can the symptomatic person's response to being diagnosed be to adapt to the role of the "sickly one" within the context of family stories? Can another family member embrace the role of caregiver within the contexts of an adopted narrative, and family stories? This is not meant to suggest that diseases are not *real* but rather to analyze the impact of family stories on family members in relation to dealing with the onset of a disease. While the entire family system will be discussed, specifically, the "dance" between the chronically-ill patient and the caregiver will be highlighted.

The purpose of this chapter is to explore the interrelationship between chronic illness, family roles, and family stories. This will entail discussing the idea of stories and narratives, and the effects of family stories on family members learning certain roles, such as the role of the care giver, and the role of family therapy in helping individuals create a new story. This new story may incorporate learning to live and function with the disease or illness in a *healthier* way. In addition to an in-depth discussion of Narrative Family therapy, a brief discussion of Alternation will be included. The chapter will conclude with a case example of the Bellasera family. Please note that all names, occupations, and identifying information used in the case example have been changed for anonymity purposes. One final note, from time to time, the reader may see words italicized. This was done to convey the idea that the meaning behind these words is open to interpretation. For example, is there such a thing as a *fact*, or do we interpret our reality as a *fact*, and thus give it meaning as such? The comedian Lily Tomlin once stated that, *reality* is a collective hunch.

The terms illness and disease are sometimes used interchangeably but there is a distinct difference in their meaning. Disease refers to a physical or psychological condition. It is a recognition that the body and/or the mind, as it may be a combination of both, are not working properly. The onset of a physical disease may also cause the onset of a psychological disease. When individuals are diagnosed with a life-threatening disease such as cancer, they often go into a depression, which is further exacerbated by grieving over the loss of their health, and the things they were once able to do but cannot do any longer. Illness, on the other hand, refers to the individual and social recognition that the condition is a problem (Kallen, 2004, p. 158). The difference between the two terms is both cultural and social. Chronic illness is not only an individual subjective experience but it takes place and has meaning within a social context. The meaning that an individual gives to the illness is influenced by his/her family of origin and on a broader level, this in turn is influenced by the social world. One's culture and social networks can shape the individual's experiences. As Rolland (2005) notes, "Families' experiences of illness are primarily influenced by the dominant culture and the larger health systems embedded in it" (p. 493). Illness-related behaviors emerge within the family context, that context co-evolves with the chronically-ill person's behavior. The behavior of the family members and the ill person become mutually maintaining over time (Vetere, 1994).

The consequences of an illness can include stigmatization due to disfigurement or the social unacceptability of the condition, the creation of stress within the family system, and the social and psychological stresses, which are a result of the cost of treatment and hospitalization. A chronic illness is persistent and ongoing. The individual usually suffers for a long period of time, often characterized by intermittent flare-ups. Frequent chronic illnesses discussed in this context include depression, asthma, and rheumatoid arthritis. Can a chronic illness, then, such as depression be a result of learned helplessness? As Gergen (1991) notes, "If we are rational creatures, we pay attention to the world and adjust our actions accordingly, thus, human actions must largely result from happenings in the social world. In short, it is not by virtue of hereditary that we are who we are, but by observation of the environment" (p.41).

Miller and Reitner (1996) suggest that a learned helplessness can be induced by specific environmental events. Depression has biological, psychological, and social symptoms that can be treated both by medication and social relearning—this is where family therapy can come into play. This will be explored in further detail, later in the chapter. Hurvitz and Straus (1991) claim that a chronically-ill person may use his/her condition to gain sympathy or maintain leverage over other family members. If a child learns that being ill comes with its own set of rewards, then the rewarded behavior serves as a reinforcer to be ill. Children may often see adults get certain rights, privileges, and attention they would not ordinarily get and this may be seen as a reward. Keeping in mind that learning and the process of socialization is a lifelong process, this may be true for adults as well.

The chronically-ill person may come to discover that his/her condition may bring with it certain rewards and attention, as well as freeing him/her from obligations. In fact, the chronically-ill individual may be the person with the most amount of power in the family system. The system begins to revolve around the person and his/her needs. Others abandon their plans, and even their own lives to care for the sick person. The reward is the non-tangible reward of power. The label of "you're the sickly one," can become a tag line and a reward. When it is time to do chores, the sickly one experiences the onset of a recurrence of the symptoms. These may then become less severe when the chores are done. The next bout, recurrence, or flare-up might not occur again, until the next time there are chores to be done.

As Rolland (2005) points out, families draw from prior multigenerational experiences with illness and loss. They use core family values to guide them. These can also designate the roles of sick members. In every family, individual members have their assigned roles. These roles can be assigned by gender, birth order, or a number of other variables, including family stories. These roles are made whether or not the designated person is well-cast for his/ her role. What determines these roles then is not based on the individual or who (s)he may be, but who the family needs them to be (Stone, 1988).

People tell stories about everything, including illness. In fact, we only know the world through the stories we make of it. Stories are central devices in the construction of human self and meaning. They anchor and explain families and their beginnings. They often act as models telling us what we should fear, avoid, or challenge. Family stories send potent messages concerning admired behaviors and preferred solutions in times of crisis and transitions.

> Stories and myths help us to order the world, to sort out, explain and integrate events in a striving for continuity and coherence; they are social touch stones mediating a complex cybernetic feedback process between the personal and the social, meshing one's inner and outer history. (Laird, 1991, p. 435)

As Gergen and Gergen (1983) note, not only do our historical accounts vary, but our versions of time itself are shaped by the stories by which we live. Through the constructions of our biographies, we recover our identities, we recollect and re-collect our own existence, our very selfhood is dependent upon the possibilities of constructing a biography. "All children in all families stumble into their designated roles, but through family stories they are coached and encouraged, and they often grow into the costume so that it becomes a second skin" (Stone, 1988, p. 87).

There are arenas where the family has its own set of rules, whether they are covert or overt, they are to be followed. Illness is one of these arenas. Illness, the role of the ill person, and the role of the caregiver become a covert form of family loyalty. This may mean that someone has to take on the role of a sick person, so that another family member can play out his or her role of the caretaker. These two enter into a collaborative dance. This dance was danced in previous generations and handed down in the form of family stories. The message may be hidden in the story but it is still present, and the dancers take their cues from it.

As children grow and develop, they tend to take on as their own, the needs and expectations that other people have of them, particularly the people who are important to them, and those that are the most emotionally close to them.

> For better or for worse, and whether we collaborate with our families or not, we are shaped by our families' notion of our identities, particularly that part of our identities which exists as an idea beyond the reach of measurement. The image they mirror back to us exists earlier and more substantially than we ourselves do. And among the primary vehicles families use to mirror us to ourselves are the family stories we hear about ourselves. These stories,… are a record of our family's fantasies, often unconscious, about who they hope we are or fear we are.
>
> The power of these fantasies and not their accuracy, is what ensures their survival. These stories … tint or taint our deepest and most intractable sense of being. (Stone, 1988. pp. 167-168)

It is the power of the fantasies and not their accuracy that count. Our deepest sense of our self and who we are is much more a matter of these stories and fantasies than of *fact*. So much so that when fantasies and *fact* collide with one another, it is easier for one to alter the *fact* to accord with the fantasy than to change the fantasy to fit the *fact*. Berger (1963) asserts this same theme in his discussion of alternation and relativization. Alternation is the reconstruction of our past to fit our present identity. This identity is continually formulated by our family of origin as well as other primary groups, and the stories and fantasies, which accompany them. One can give meaning to past events or strip it away, based on one's concept of self. A self that is ultimately social in process and continually evolving. As such it is important to remember that our past is resided in our memory. But memory is not a constant. It is malleable and open to interpretation. Berger's (1963) point is that we remember those things that are important to us and that support our present identity. These memories are given importance today, an importance they may not have had when they happened. We tend to think of memory as a recorder or a camera where the past is filed and can be called up at will. In *truth,* memory is a story teller. It creates and shapes meaning by emphasizing some things and leaving other things out. When memory speaks it tells a narrative *truth,* which has more influence than historical accuracy. The *facts* that clients tell the therapist are partly historical and partly constructions (Nichols & Schwartz, 2007). Narrative family therapy reminds us that problem stories are not personal failings, but stories of domination, alienation, and frustration. Narrative family therapists help the family members to search their memories for the other side of the story—the side that honors their courage and persistence, the side that opens the way for hope (Nichols & Schwartz, 2006). In so doing, narrative family therapists enable their clients to create new stories about themselves, new memories, and new identities.

There is a special form of family stories known as family myths. Family myths, like classical myths are meant to explain why. They offer possible, if not always plausible, explanations within the family (Stone, 1988). Family myths deal in code with the important human issues of birth, death, sexuality, injury, and illness. The family myths include the identified roles of its members. The family myth explains the behavior of the individuals in the family while it hides its motives. The beliefs, which serve as the foundation of the myth preserve the family's homeostasis. This is the case even if one member has to bear a socially stigmatized role such as "the bad one" or "the black sheep," "the sickly one," or "the ill one."

Through the telling of family stories and the preservation of family myths, and their covert and overt messages, and behaviors of the family, children can learn a great deal about being ill. They can learn that being sick is one way of guaranteeing that one is taken care of; that one can get out of chores; and that rewards may be forthcoming. Illness can be a reliable and appropriate way of getting needed attention. "A good parent is someone who takes care of a sick child and a child is someone who ought to be sick in order to demonstrate that the parent is a good parent" (Stone, 1988, pp. 80-81). Likewise, a good child is someone who takes care of a sick parent and a parent is someone who ought to be sick in order to demonstrate that the child is a good child. Patterns of coping with illness are transmitted across generations as are family myths, taboos, catastrophic events, and belief systems (Rolland, 2005).

Illness in a family can be used to blame someone or as a method of retaliation as in, "I'm sick. It's your fault. You are to blame." In other families, sickness is permitted to some members but denied to others. This allows the family to be dichotomized between those who are "afflicted" and those who are the "survivors" (Stone, 1988).

"Family stories, whatever else they are, can be little moments of history or slices of sociology" (Stone, 1988, p. 243). As to our sense of self and our biographies, family stories offer us our own mentor, in that they willingly give us our roles as to who we are to be in our families. Just as our sense of self is always in process and always in flux, so too are our biographies. They are always in a state of being revised. One's biography is so much more than just what happened in one's life. It is essentially a view of oneself from a certain perspective or lens at a certain point in time. Given this perspective, certain *facts* become irrelevant if they do not fit with our sense of self. Other *facts* are accorded great importance because they support one's vision of one's self and thus fit into one's autobiography. This is what Berger (1963) meant in his discussion of alternation. One's autobiography or one's stories of one's life are told in narrative form. It is important to remark that narratives are socially constructed through a number of factors.

The narrator will tell the story through what Mills (1940) would call a "Vocabulary of Motives." Mills makes the point that meanings are socially situated and identifies one as a member of a specific group, in this case the family. In narratives, individuals are seen as organizing their experience in the form of stories. Stories, then, become a context in which certain information fits but other information does not. Personal narratives are not neutral. They are told from the position and perspective of self as narrator. A consequence of this is a meaning-making process about the others involved. Since one usually experiences one's own intention as good, then the problem is seen as stemming from the other's actions and the other's intentions (as less than pure).

Narratives on a broad definitional sense are relevant to every level of human experience, and social organization. As Laird (1991) points out, to understand or interpret a narrative, one must understand the event structure (*facts* of the narrative), the evaluative structure (what meaning the narrator makes of the *facts*), and the explanatory structure (the speaker's worldview or belief system). The explanatory structure is the narrator's personal paradigm for making sense out of the world. In this sense, self-narrative is the individual's account of the relationship among self-relevant events across time, a way of connecting coherently the events of one's own life. Similarly, Gergen and Gergen (1983) state that as we communicate our personal narratives we subject them to social alteration or critique. As Berger (1963) would note, we alternate them. Whether or not a narrative can be maintained depends on the individual's skill in negotiating with others or convincing others that his/her interpretation of events is correct.

The narratives people construct evolve in and are unique to the social, cultural, and relational construct in which they are constructed and in which they become maintained. One's culture, one's collectivity, one's family of origin, one's primary groups provide exemplary story models from which the individual's narrative draws shape and expression, and within which interpretation is possible, connecting the individual to the culture.

Gergen and Gergen (1983) refer to "nested-narratives." Nested-narratives means that one's biography is a collection of specific vignettes, which account for specific events, feelings, interpretations, or offer an image of self as a worthwhile moral person. These vignettes often carry very important messages to the narrator and the listener. Such a message can include, "You are to take care of me as I am ill, and you are my youngest child."

From this perspective we can view therapy as narrative-in-construction, the restorying of the couples and families who present for therapy. As Heitler (1993) points out, *reality* changes, such as the advent of chronic illness, requires families to restructure themselves to adapt to new conditions. A narrative assessment consists of getting the family's story. This is not just meant to be information gathering but it is also a reconstructive inquiry that is designed to move clients to the belief that they have some power over their problems.

Family rules and family stories can be discovered in therapy in genograms. A genogram contains all the salient *facts* as told in stories about nuclear and extended families including dates (birth, marriages, divorces, deaths) of *significant* events, illnesses, etc. The genogram can reveal patterns that have governed the family for a number of generations (usually three or four). The genogram gives the therapist a picture of the clients' families through the eyes of the client. It has been constructed by the client in part, from the family stories that the client knows.

When one thinks genogram, one thinks Bowen (1978). From a Bowenian point of view, symptoms can show up in one of three locations: in the marital relationship in the form of distance, conflict, or divorce; in the health of one of the partners; or in one of the children (Bowen, 1978). The couple that is discussed in the case study, James and Connie Bellasera were asked to construct genograms. It was through the discussion of the genograms that the meaning of family stories in their lives became most poignant.

Life is complicated so we find ways to explain it. These explanations, the stories we tell ourselves organize our experience and shape our behavior. The stories that are told to us and that we in turn tell ourselves are powerful because they determine what we notice and remember, and therefore how we face the future. "… The narrative metaphor focuses on self-defeating cognitions—the stories people tell themselves about their problems…. The narrative metaphor … focuses on expanding clients' thinking to allow them to consider alternative ways of looking at themselves and their problems" (Nichols & Schwartz, 2006, p. 338).

Narrative family therapy is consistent with postmodernism and social constructionism. The narrative family therapist views him/herself as a collaborator and thus assumes a non-expert stance. As such, the narrative family therapist becomes a questioner who finds unique outcomes or exceptions. The narrative family therapist assists the family in separating themselves from old, problem-saturated stories by constructing new stories in which they, instead of the problem, are in control (Gladdings, 2007). The narrative approach is built around two organizing metaphors: personal narrative and social construction (Nichols & Schwartz, 2007). The narrative family therapy perspective is that people live their lives by their stories (Kurtz & Tandy, 1995). "Families are formed, perpetuated, and transformed through the stories they share" (Ponzetti, 2005, p.132).

The narrative approach in family therapy is exemplified in the works of Michael White and David Epston (1991). Their approach emphasizes narrative reasoning, which is portrayed in the telling of stories. Narrative reasoning helps families generate alternative stories to their lives in order to come up with novel options and strategies. In particular White (1986, 1989, 1992, 1993, 1995) sees people's problems as related to the stories they have of themselves, which often reflect cultural practices. These cultural practices can sometimes be very oppressive. The emphasis in narrative family therapy is towards a story line way of conceptualizing and interpreting the world. It emphasizes empowering families to develop their own unique and alternative stories about themselves. Narrative reasoning can help families generate alternative stories to their history, and thus come up with novel options and strategies for living their lives. By re-authoring their lives families become empowered to change (White, 1995).

In narrative family therapy problems are seen as oppressive, and therefore eliminated as quickly as possible. Problem-saturated stories encourage people to respond to each other in ways that perpetuate the problem story. The family members' responses to each other become invitations to more of the same and further support the hardening and entrenchment of problem stories. The therapist assists families in separating themselves from old, problem-saturated stories by constructing new stories in which they are in control. This is what is often referred to as "re-authoring" (Gladdings, 2007). It involves the defining of lives and relationships in new narratives. Clients are helped to move beyond symptom maintaining myths, and taken-for-granted *realities*, to construct a new, more vital story. Re-authoring allows families to change in new and different ways; in ways not previously thought possible (White, 1995). Clients change their lives by changing their stories.

The narrative approach also distinguishes between logico-scientific reasoning characterized by empiric and logic; and narrative reasoning, which is characterized by stories, substories, meaningfulness, and liveliness. Narrative therapy recognized that stories do not just mirror life, but in fact, they shape it. "That's why people have the interesting habit of becoming the stories they tell about their experience ... by delving into people's stories, narrative therapists are able to understand and influence what makes them act as they do" (Nichols & Schwartz, 2007, p. 264).

Narrative therapy is viewed as encouraging clients to:

- take a collaborative, empathic position with strong interest in a client's story;
- search for times in a client's history when he /she was strong and resourceful;
- use questions to take a non-imposing, respectful approach to any new story put forth;
- to never label people but instead treat them as human beings with unique personal histories; and
- help people separate from the dominant cultural narratives they have internalized so as to open space for alternative life stories (White, 1995).

The strategies of narrative therapy fall into three stages: first, the problem narrative stage, which involves recasting the problem as an affliction by focusing on its effects rather than its causes. This is also known as externalizing the problem. Second, by finding exceptions which consist of past triumphs over the problem. Times when the family did not succumb to the influence of the problem. Finally, the recruitment of support. Encouraging celebrations or public rituals reinforce new and preferred interpretations, and moves cognitive construction into socially-supported action (Nichols & Schwartz, 2007).

Narrative family therapy involves a number of treatment techniques. These techniques will be briefly discussed. Externalization (White & Epston, 1991) allows the problem to become a separate entity from the client. The problem is no longer viewed as something that is personal to one or more members of the family but rather it is viewed as a problem the family needs to solve together because of its negative impact on the family. Ideally, the family forms a teams and enters into a dialogue about problem solving. Thus, there no longer is an identified patient but rather a family system working against the common enemy.

The influence or effect of the problem on the person asks each family member how the problem has influenced him/ her in an effort to increase his/her objectivity and awareness (White & Epston, 1991). The therapist asks each family member to give a detailed no-holds barred account of how the problem has affected him/her. For example, "How has *the problem* influenced you and your life, and your relationships?" (Gladdings, 2007). Similarly, the therapist asks about the influence or the effect of the person on the problem. Asking family members how they have influenced a problem makes them increasingly aware of their response to a problem, while simultaneously helping them to realize their strengths in facing the situation (White & Epston, 1991).

Raising dilemmas and predicting setbacks (White, 1986) are two strategies that are used especially after the family has made some movement toward creating new stories around the problem. Raising dilemmas allows families to examine possible aspects of a problem before the need arises. The family is asked how they would cope with the problem if it became better, worsened, or remained the same. As setbacks are bound to happen, narrative family therapists view setbacks as best dealt with when they are planned for and anticipated. Families then have the opportunity to decide ahead of time how they will act in the face of a setback. The question is basically, "What would the family do if the resolved problem were to re-occur?" (Gladdings, 2007).

Therapists can challenge families to examine the nature of the difficulties they bring to therapy and what resources they have at their disposal and can use to handle their problem through the use of questions. Narrative family therapy is about asking questions. The questions include exception questions, which are directed towards finding instances when the problem did not occur; and significance questions, which are unique redescription questions (Kurtz & Tandy, 1995). Significance questions search for and reveal the meanings, significance, and importance of the exceptions. Exception questions often begin with "when" or "what." They can also be phrased in such a way as to get the family to remember the exception. For example, "Was there ever a time when ...?"

Letters serve as a continuation of the dialogue between the therapist and the family. They are also reminders of what occurred in the therapy sessions. Epston (1994) frequently uses letters in his therapy with his clients. "Words in a letter don't fade or disappear the way a conversation does.... A client can hold a letter in hand, reading and rereading it days, months, and years after the session" (p. 31).

An effective way to end therapy with a client family is through celebrations and certificates. Celebrations and certificates (White & Epston, 1991) are tangible affirmations that the problem has been defeated. They also mark the beginning of a new description of the family.

Narrative family therapists do therapy by constantly posing questions to their clients. It is a question oriented therapy. Packaging interventions in the form of questions makes it seem less like advice that can be resisted and challenged by the client(s), and more like forming a partnership with the client family. As such narrative therapists employ a variety of questions which include: deconstruction questions which focus on externalizing the problem; opening space questions which uncover the unique outcomes; preference questions which ensure that unique outcomes represent preferred experiences; story development questions encourage the client family to develop a new story from the unique outcomes; meaning questions challenge negative images of self; and questions that extend the story into the future help to support changes and reinforce positive developments (Nichols & Schwartz, 2006).

Case Study: the Bellasera Family

James (50) and Connie (45) Bellasera presented for couple therapy after being married for approximately three years. Their marriage was preceded by a rather long courtship period. They had dated for close to five years, and then had been engaged for another two before they married. James was the youngest of six children, and the only male. He and his siblings were all very close in age, in that there was only two years between each birth. There was one set of twins. His father had died shortly before he began dating Connie. James was a tax attorney and was successfully established in his own practice before they married. Shortly after his father died, James purchased a two family house where he lived with his mother, Nancy. His mother occupied the first floor apartment, and James had the second floor. James had never been married before and was the only single sibling when he and Connie married.

Connie was the eldest of four children. She had a younger brother, and two younger sisters. One of her sisters and her brother were both married with children. The youngest sister was a lesbian and had been living with her partner for nine years. Connie's mother was alive and living in a private townhouse in a senior community. Connie's father had died about two months after she had married James. Connie taught English in a middle school and was also the coach for the girls' swimming team. This was Connie's second marriage. She had been married to her first husband for only two years when he left her for another woman. Connie had married her first husband when she was 25, and they were divorced shortly before her 29th birthday. They had not had any children. In the years between her divorce and meeting James, Connie had dated rarely and not at all seriously. After her divorce, Connie had moved back in with her parents for a little over a year, but then moved into her own apartment (despite her parents' protests). She had moved back in with her parents after she and James had become engaged, and had remained there until they married.

The problem that brought them into therapy was that Connie and James were arguing a great deal about his relationship with his mother. Although as Connie put it, "We are the only couple I know who whispers when they argue lest she (referring to Nancy) not hear us." Connie and James had moved into his house, and his second floor apartment when they married. Connie was not in favor of this arrangement and this was one of the main reasons they had had such a long courtship. She had finally "given in" to James, and was regretful of her decision.

Connie described James as a loving son, brother, and husband (she seemed to be highlighting the order in which she described his roles) but felt he was too involved with his mother, and to a lesser extent his sisters. James described Connie as a loving wife who was very sincere and considerate. He felt that Connie was very close to her family as well; and had an especially close relationship with her youngest sister. James also noted that Connie was the only woman of the many women that he had dated that his mother liked. This was surprising to him, since his mother usually disapproved of the women he dated.

When James was about twenty years old, his parents had been in a rather serious car accident. While his father sustained minor injuries including cuts, bruises, and two broken fingers, it was his mother who was more seriously hurt. She had suffered a number of broken bones, including a fractured pelvis. After a lengthy recuperation in the hospital, she had spent years in physical therapy. She was able to walk but her gait was slow and unsteady. She often complained of great pain in her legs. The family referred to these episodes as "flare-ups." When Connie and James entered therapy, Nancy was eighty-one years old.

Her flare-ups had become more debilitating and more frequent as she aged. She was able to function but at times she had her "bad days." Occasionally, the pain and discomfort would become so severe that Nancy would confine herself to a wheel chair for a period of time. Despite her illness, Nancy and James' father had continued to travel extensively and entertain frequently, as they had done when James and his sisters were growing up. They were often cared for by James' paternal grandmother until she died when James was thirteen years old. After that, when his parents traveled he was often watched by his older sisters.

James paid for his mother to have a certified nurse assistant every night, and a cleaning lady who came four times a week. She was part cleaning lady and part companion. Even though James' father had left Nancy rather financially secure when he died, she had spent a great deal of money on herself. Within the last few years, James had to help his mother to continue to live the life to which she was accustomed. Nancy was a demanding woman who expected a great deal from her children, especially her only son. She expected total loyalty, and she expected her children to be there when she needed them. She expected all of her children to care for her, but much more was expected from James, since he was the youngest.

When Nancy experienced a flare-up, the lives of her children stopped and her every whim was catered to. The situation was made worse when Nancy was diagnosed with depression after James' father died. After his death, Nancy began experiencing more flare-ups, and became increasingly isolated. This added to her depression, and her dependence on James. Her depression also caused more flare-ups, which further isolated her and increased James' role as her caretaker. A vicious cycle of depression, flare-ups, isolation, and James as caretaker was beginning to dominate their lives and their relationship. Over the past ten years, Nancy had demanded more of her children, especially James. Nancy's last flare-up, which had occurred three months before James and Connie came into therapy, had been one of her worse. It had caused James and Connie to cancel their vacation, the first one they had planned to take since their honeymoon. Connie claimed that while she knew that Nancy was sick, her condition was a tool that she used to control her children, especially James.

It was clear that Nancy's illness was her most powerful tool and a mechanism she used to control her children and keep them at her side. When Nancy would experience a severe flare-up, she would confine herself to the wheelchair. All her children would rush over and care to her needs including taking her to the doctor and for therapy (both emotional and physical). Vacations and parties were cancelled until Nancy felt better, and was able to attend. As Nancy's condition would stabilize and things calmed down, her children would resume their *normal* lives. Nancy would feel ignored and another flare-up would occur. As much as Nancy demanded their attention and total devotion when she experienced a flare-up, she always had a miraculous recovery when it meant her going out, or away with friends. Connie believed that Nancy used her illness to control the lives of her children, especially James. James was disappointed with Connie's "inconsiderate attitude" as anyone could see that his mother was ill.

During an early therapy session, James had commented that his grandmother (Nancy's mother) had been diagnosed with a heart murmur when Nancy was about sixteen. Nancy had spent most of her teenage years and early adulthood caring for her mother. Nancy was the youngest of six children and the only one that was still living at home when this happened. When Nancy and James' father had married, Nancy took her mother to live with them until she died a few years later. Nancy and James' father had been in Ohio visiting his family when Nancy's mother had the fatal attack. As James commented to Connie, "This is what families do, take care of each other."

As therapy progressed with James and Connie it became clear that the stories of illness in James' family were central to its individuals' sense of self, and central to the family as a whole. Family stories may not easily encompass intricate explanations of the many causes for an event. In fact, they serve to reduce complex phenomena to a single comprehensible cause. Why does James care for his mother to the extent he does? Simply, because Nancy as the youngest did it for her mother. A family's current behavior cannot be adequately comprehended apart from its history. This is especially true for families that face a chronic illness (Rolland, 2005).

This is what James and the rest of the Bellasera siblings did when Nancy became ill. The family story was clear, that the youngest was to take care of the sick mother. James embraced the role and gave himself a narrative of good son within the family story that good children take care of their ill parents. In therapy, it is paramount that James and Connie construct a new story for themselves as a couple, and new narratives for themselves as individuals.

At the end of the second session with James and Connie they were asked to separately construct a genogram of their families of origin. In the third session they were discussed, and it was then that the story of illness in Connie's family was revealed. Illness in Connie's family was defined differently than it was in James' family. Connie, like James, is of Italian descent, but her family is from "the heel of the boot," or Sicily. Connie's genogram depicted five generations beginning with her great grandparents and ending with her nieces and nephews. Growing up, Connie and her siblings were closer to her father's side of the family (the Rizzo family). While Connie did not know her great grandparents, she recounts with fondness the stories her paternal grandmother, "Nana Maria," told her. The first story involves Nana Maria's father, Paolo. Paolo owned a donkey and a cart, and he made his living by transporting people, and things for businesses from one town to another (part taxi cab and trucking service). On this one day, Paolo and his son, Nino, were returning from delivering items to a nearby town. They stopped to eat lunch and unhitched the donkey from the cart so that it could freely graze. When they had finished their lunch and were ready to begin their journey again, Paolo and Nino tried to hitch the donkey back up to the cart. As donkeys can be stubborn, the donkey decided it was not finished eating its lunch. As they tried to hitch the donkey, it became very angry and began to kick. It kicked Nino in the head and he died instantly. As Paolo bent over his son to see what had happened to him, the donkey kicked him in the backside causing him to lurch forward. Paolo was thrown to the grown and knocked unconscious. When Paolo woke up he placed his dead son on the cart, hitched the donkey, made his last delivery, and returned home. It was Nana Maria's belief that her father had sustained a serious concussion because from this point forward, Paolo began to suffer from constant and severe headaches. Even though Paolo woke up every morning with a headache, he continued to work. Nana Maria recounts the story noting that her father never missed a day of work. In fact, he died while on the job.

One morning, Paolo woke up with an unusually bad headache, and his wife begged him to stay home and rest. Nonetheless, he and his brother went to work. They were on their way to deliver some grain to a nearby town when, according to Paolo's bother, he began to grip his head in pain, he collapsed, and died. His brother still went to make the delivery, and then returned to their village with Paolo dead in the cart.

The second story involves Nana Maria, herself. She and her husband, Maurizio, owned a small fruit and vegetable store. Maurizio employed a neighbor's son to make deliveries to the neighbors. However, he was lazy, and tended not to be very reliable. He would often take the store bicycle to deliver an order to a neighbor a few blocks away, and then not return for hours. Nana Maria was pregnant with Connie's father at the time. This one day the delivery boy did not show up to work, as usual, so Maurizio had to make the deliveries himself. It was a hot August day, and Nana Maria was due to give birth any day but she went to the store and was working behind the counter when suddenly she went into labor.

A customer called the midwife, and summoned Maurizio home. Nana Maria went into the back room, gave birth to her third child and her second son, and then went back to work. However, during the birth, she had lost a lot of blood. Maurizio seeing how pale and tired she looked, told her to stay in bed but she knew that he had to make the deliveries and with three children, they needed to keep the business running. The next morning as she was tending the counter, she passed out. Maurizio summoned the doctor who told Nana Maria she needed to rest, but as she would say to Connie, "We come from Palermo and strong Sicilian blood pulses through our veins. No doctor was going to keep me and your grandfather from working and feeding our children. So, that night I made a big pot of lentil soup for dinner and the next day I was fine." In Connie's family, illness was dismissed. It never interfered with work, and work was paramount to everything else including socializing.

James and Connie told a number of stories in the therapy sessions. These stories also served to justify their assumptions about the beliefs they held in regards to their own families of origin, and to each others' families. These stories had editors. For James the editor of the Bellasera family was often his mother. For Connie, the editor of the Rizzo family was her paternal grandmother, Nana Maria. Horton and Andonian (2005) speak of family stories as metaphors, noting the importance of the editor. The editor is the person who determines what stories are told, whose voice gets heard, and when it is heard. As the editor, this person sets "editorial policy." "While editors are not necessary for multiple stories to exist, they can play a role in encouraging or discouraging voice, interpreting stories, giving weight or emphasis to some stories or aspects thereof, or shaping and accommodating multiple truths within the family anthology" (Horton & Andonian, 2005, p.89). The editor can then determine which stories get told, and the meaning of the story. The editor can also downplay alternative meanings.

James and Connie both accepted the stories told in their families by their respective editors. The story in James' family was that illness was acceptable, that the sick person must be cared for, and that the one who did the caring was the youngest child. This story seemed to override gender. In Connie's family, death, let alone illness, did not stop family members from going to work, and accomplishing what needed to be done. Even though sick family members did not expect to be taken care of, when someone in the family tried to assume the role of caretaker, that person was dismissed. It is interesting to note the editorial policy that Nana Maria put on the story of her father's death. Her mother had asked Paolo not to go to work but he did, and he died. The emphasis could have been that not listening caused his death; it could have been that men should listen to their wives lest tragedy befall them; or it could have been that men are stubborn. The meaning Nana Maria made and shared with Connie is that of strength, of doing what needed to be done to take care of your family. Nana Maria, likewise, had not heeded her husband's advice not to return to work after she gave birth. While she had not died, she had only fainted. Who was the antagonist in the story, it was the delivery boy who was described as lazy and therefore unreliable. Nana Maria was also adding a meaning about family and roles within the family. It is the duty of parents to take care of their children, versus the duty of children to take care of their parents, and this is paramount over everything else, including one's health and to some extent, one's life.

The role of therapy was to have the stories of the Bellasera and Rizzo families coexist and for Connie and James to create new narratives and new family stories. It was also to help them construct a meaning around these old family stories, a meaning that would suit them as a couple. The postmodern perspective in family therapy creates a therapeutic system that allows this to occur. The work of narrative therapists have made some of the most significant contributions to the appreciation of language, story, and metaphor that is a hallmark of postmodern family therapy, and that has become second nature to family therapists today (Hoffman, 2002). It thus seemed that the most likely way to proceed with James and Connie was through a narrative family therapy lens.

While the presenting problem that James and Connie began therapy with was their arguing about his relationship with Nancy and her illness, it became clear that the issue was deeper. In an early session, James and Connie were asked to face each other and express their concerns to each other in the form of "I" statements. James commented that he felt misunderstood when Connie did not support and consider his sense of deep responsibility for his family of origin. Connie stated that she felt unloved and unvalued when James put his responsibility to his family above his responsibility to her. They were then asked to think about the message they both had received from their families of origin concerning responsibility. James noted that it was his responsibility to be the caregiver in the family. Connie stated that responsibility for her meant to care for one's family. To Connie, this was the most important responsibility one had in life. Thus, they came to realize that their ideas about responsibility to one's family were not so far apart. White (1986, 1989, 1992, 1993, 1995) views people's problems as related to the stories they have of themselves, which may reflect cultural practices. Both James and Connie were Italian-Americans who had internalized the role of responsibility for family into their own life story.

Narrative reasoning can help families generate alternative stories to their history, and thus come up with novel options and strategies for living their lives. By re-authoring their lives, family members are increasingly empowered to change (Gladdings, 2007). Could James change the role of caregiver to Nancy? Could he re-author this dominant role in his life? What can Connie do to aid James in this process? In what ways may she have to re-author aspects and roles in her life?

Connie noted that she realized that James had long been the caregiver to Nancy but felt that he had enabled his mother's condition, and she was using it to dominate their relationship. James was asked how he felt about being given the role of caregiver. He said it was a difficult role, one he had never really wanted, and one he found himself increasingly disliking. He felt that while his sisters did help him, all of the major responsibility fell on him. He made all of the important decisions regarding Nancy's health care. It was a powerful responsibility and he was afraid that if he left Nancy during one of her flare-ups (reminiscent of the story of his grandmother's death. Nancy and James' father were away when her mother sustained the fatal heart attack), his sisters would blame him, and he would feel guilty for the rest of his life.

From White's (1989, 1993) perspective, families feel oppressed by symptomatic behavior. His therapy is aimed at getting family members to unite and take back control of their lives from the oppressive symptoms. Both James and Connie were feeling oppressed against his caregiving responsibilities. Having them take back control, James and Connie would come to view themselves as a healthy unit struggling against a troublesome externalized problem, his caregiving responsibility. It would enable them to deconstruct the old story, and reconstruct a new more empowering one.

Narrative reasoning emphasizes externalizing problems in order to solve them. Here, the problem becomes a separate entity. James and Connie could reduce their arguing over his caregiving responsibilities by forming a team, and beginning a new dialogue about solving the problem. By externalizing the problem, Connie and James could allow for new possibilities, and feel less stressed in approaching problems. In externalization the problem can be described in such a way that it takes on a personality of its own. It was decided that caregiving responsibilities should be given a nickname (White, 1989).

James and Connie were asked to come up with a nickname for James' caregiving responsibilities. In the next session, Connie announced with some excitement that they had come up with a nickname, they were going to call it "brutta cosa" (an Italian phrase, which when translated into English means a bad or ugly thing). It was agreed that from that day forward, James' caregiving responsibility would be called and referred to as brutta cosa. James' caregiving responsibilities has now been redefined into an objectified, reified, external tyrant with a will of its own. James and Connie can now be asked to come together against brutta cosa. James and Connie were also asked if there were other people in their lives who could help them in their battle against brutta cosa. James and Connie both mentioned that they supposed his sisters could help, and to a lesser extent her mother and siblings. It was agreed, although somewhat hesitantly by James, as he was holding on to his role of caregiver, that they would talk with his sisters and see if they were able to join them in a therapy session.

Narrative family therapy believes that the self is constituted in social interaction. Narrative therapists make a point of helping clients find an audience to support their progress in constructing new stories for themselves. James and Connie were being asked to contact people who can help them construct and authenticate their new story. James and Connie were being asked to recruit people in their lives who can serve as supportive witnesses of their new story. First, it was the Bellasera family. Later the Rizzo family would also be called upon to support their new story and new identities.

During the week, Connie called to state that his sisters were willing to come to help them out, although the eldest sister was the most resistant. When James and Connie arrived with his sisters a few weeks later, they had already explained to them why they had come into therapy. James began the session by explaining what brutta cosa was, and that his caregiving responsibilites with Nancy were to be referred to by this new name. There were more than a few raised eyebrows, but they were willing to try. The session then concentrated on their responses to some of the following questions: "How has brutta cosa influenced you and your relationship with your siblings?"; "How has brutta cosa affected your relationships with your spouses and your children?"; and "How has brutta cosa affected your relationship with Nancy?" This technique allowed the family to gain distance from the problem and to detach from the dominant story line. Additionally, it did not seem to his sisters that James and Connie were attacking Nancy and her illness. In fact, her name was only mentioned a few times. James' sisters did not have to feel defensive about protecting themselves or their mother as it was brutta cosa who was the trouble maker. By the end of the session they had engaged in a rather lively dialogue about the affects of brutta cosa in their lives, and had even had a few laughs over brutta cosa. Connie, James, and his sisters had already begun to deconstruct the old story, and were beginning to reconstruct a new story about their relationship to each other and their mother.

Much to James and Connie's surprise, two of his sisters had felt that Nancy was manipulating them all by her flare-ups. They had noticed that this happened when she was feeling ignored and seemed to get better when it was time for Nancy to go out with her family and friends. They began to realize that perhaps her isolation was contributing to the frequency and duration of the flare-ups. They all agreed that James had been the primary caretaker and understood the burden that brutta cosa had put on him and his relationship with Connie. His eldest sister had noted that on more than one occasion she had felt a little resentful that James had "taken on" brutta cosa because she felt that as the eldest daughter some of that responsibility should have been hers. His sisters were also surprised to hear that he did not like brutta cosa, as it was their opinion that he had freely taken on the role. At the end of the session, the eldest sister said to James, "Jimbo (the sisters' nickname for their baby brother), you can rely on us to help you because that is what families do, help each other. Anytime you begin to feel that brutta cosa is invading your life, you call us and we, together as a family, will help you and Connie to throw it in the 'bunkulaura.'" They explained that this term referred to a slang word for bathtub in their family. They said that growing up when they were a bit mischievous, their father would playfully tell them that if they did not behave and stop their "horsing around," he was going to throw them into the "bunkulaura." Over the years they had thrown many things in the "bunkulaura" including scary things in the night, old boy or girl friends who had broken their hearts, and a few other private things. Each had used the bunkulaura at one point in time as their personal dumping ground for the hurts of life.

The Bellaseras were now being presented with a non-pathological view of the problem, brutta cosa, one in which no one was to blame. They were offered the opportunity to co-construct with the therapist a new narrative that provided an alternate account of their lives. Two processes were simultaneously happening: deconstruction and reconstruction (White, 1992). The Bellasera family was free to deconstruct the history of brutta cosa and some of their old stories that had shaped their lives, and reconstruct a new story with a new way of being.

James, Connie, and his sisters returned to therapy together for another session or two. Dilemmas were raised to the family so that they could examine aspects of brutta cosa or another problem before it arose. It was important to include James' sisters since they were essential in helping Connie and James defeat brutta cosa. It was also important that someone else would not adopt brutta cosa. They were intent on ridding their lives of brutta cosa.

A dilemma that was raised was Nancy's reaction to James letting go of brutta cosa. Nancy would most likely feel a sense of disloyalty from James, and would become angry with him, or more likely Connie. Also, Nancy might begin to experience more frequent and lengthier flare-ups in an effort to ensnare James into taking care of her, and thus allowing brutta cosa to reappear. As much as James wanted to give up brutta cosa, he might be resistant to it as well.

Since setbacks are bound to happen, narrative family therapy takes the approach that this inevitability is best dealt with when it is planned (White, 1986). Families then can decide ahead of time how they will act in the face of adversity. What would the Bellasera family do if brutta cosa reappeared the next time Nancy had a flare-up? Would they allow brutta cosa in or would they fight back and drive it away again? How could they get rid of brutta cosa permanently? Through the use of such questions, the family is challenged in therapy to look at the resources they possess.

The family was also asked about exceptions to the problem, or unique outcomes. These questions reveal the meanings, the significance, and the importance of exceptions. "Unique outcomes open room for counterplots, new and more empowering ways of constructing events.... These newly attended to times of effectiveness provide openings around which to weave a new and more optimistic story" (Nichols & Schwartz, 2006, P. 344). Connie and James were asked if there were times in the past when they had not succumbed to brutta cosa, and what had happened? James noted that the previous summer he and Connie had gone for the weekend (Connie noted that it was only one night, from Saturday afternoon to Sunday afternoon) to visit Connie's sister at the summer place she and her partner owned on Fire Island. They had just boarded the boat when his beeper went off, and he noticed it was Nancy calling him. There was not a telephone on the boat (this was before everyone owned a cell phone) so he had to wait until they got to Connie's sister house. When they arrived, he immediately called Nancy who told him that she was having a flare-up and she wanted him to please come home. James had initially considered it but when he looked at the boat schedule and considered the time it would take them to drive back, he instead called his eldest sister and asked her to check in on Nancy. She called James back later in the evening, and told him that she had taken Nancy to her house to spend the night, and all was fine. She had given Nancy her medication and she was fast asleep.

The next day James and Connie had a leisurely morning and then started their trip back home. Connie remarked that she was impressed that James had not tried to contact his mother at all on Sunday. When they returned home, Nancy was still not home but there was a message from another sister that she had taken Nancy to her house for the day, they were going to go out to dinner, and then she would drop her off. When Nancy got home a few hours later, she was fine. Connie had noted to James that nothing had happened to Nancy, and "In fact, the world had not come to an end."

As James and Connie continued to drive brutta cosa out of their lives, Connie had reached out to her family, and engaged the help of the Rizzo family as well. Connie's siblings would make it a point to invite Nancy to family events (even if James and Connie could not attend) that she might enjoy. Connie's mother also suggested that Nancy visit her, and invited her to special events and outings at the senior complex. As Nancy began to be more active, as she had been prior to her husband's death, her flare-ups were happening less often, and they were less severe when they did occur. Connie's youngest sister had even invited Nancy and her mother to spend a few days with her and her partner on Fire Island. Nancy went and upon returning told James and Connie that on Saturday night they had friends over for a bar-b-que. Nancy said that she had a "wild weekend of fun." Additionally, James and Connie's families were growing closer. Nancy and Connie's mother were also becoming very good friends.

Connie and James were coming to therapy much less frequently as they had the tools to work on other issues. As for brutta cosa, it had not come around recently. They seemed prepared to terminate. "The tenacious confidence in people that narrative therapists convey with genuine respect and caring is contagious. As clients come to trust their therapist, they can borrow that confidence and use it in dealing with their problems" (Nichols & Schwartz, 2007, p. 269).

As it became clear that therapy was going to end, a celebration was planned. Celebrations and certificates are a unique and important aspect of narrative therapy. They are used to bring closure to therapy. They serve to commemorate both the defeat of the problem (brutta cosa), as well as to mark the beginning of a new family story (White & Epston, 1991). Connie and James planned a party that included their mothers, their siblings, and their spouses/partners. Everybody volunteered to bring something such as food and drink. A Certificate of Achievement was prepared and presented to James and Connie at the end of the party. It read:

> "This award is presented to
> James and Connie Bellasera
> who with the help of their families
> conquered Brutta Cosa, and replaced
> it with Bella Cosa" (beautiful thing).

The members of the Bellasera and Rizzo families were invited to sign their names at the bottom. Just as the celebration was ending, Nancy stood up and said that she had an announcement to make. She told James and Connie that they needed to find a new tenant as she had decided (with a little help from Connie's mother) to buy a condo in the same senior complex where Connie's mother lived. As she noted, "You kids are cramping my style."

All of these efforts such as the celebration and the making and signing of the certificate are useful tools for the family, and are in keeping with the social constructionist emphasis in narrative family therapy on interaction in creating and maintaining change.

The story of James and Connie Bellasera illustrates how family therapists can co-construct with their clients a new story about their lives. In this case, narrative family therapy was employed. James had to abandon his role of caregiver. He and Connie with the help of their families of origin were able to defeat brutta cosa, and in so doing they were able to empower themselves. As their roles changed, so did Nancy's. While Nancy was not miraculously cured, she too had become empowered and was able to change her role. She was now living her life with more freedom and responsibility.

Family therapists have an obligation to listen to the stories' of their clients' lives. These stories have meaning for them, and are essential to their roles in their families, and in their definitions of self. The diagnosis of a chronic illness can be a very destabilizing factor in a family. As the family begins to grapple with it, they will rely on their family history, and on family stories to help them gain balance. However, in so doing, they may be forced to adopt and embrace a role that is dysfunctional.

Family members can then become entrenched in roles that serve no one. In the hands of family therapists they are allowed to re-author the stories of their lives, they are able to deconstruct the old story of their self, and reconstruct a new empowering story.

By utilizing a narrative family therapy perspective, James and Connie were able to value their own life experiences and stories while simultaneously reconstructing and re-authoring these stories. In this process, the problems became less dominant. As James and Connie were encouraged to utilize family resources (both the Bellasera and Rizzo families), externalize the problem (brutta cosa), and expect and discuss setbacks and dilemmas, they were able to disengage themselves from a problem saturated story. They were free to rid themselves of old and unproductive patterns of perception and behavior. They were then also free to establish new stories, new ways of acting and feeling, new identities, and new relationships with each other and their families.

References

Berger, P.L. (1963). *Invitation to Sociology: A Humanistic Perspective.* Garden City, NY: Anchor Books.

Bowen, M. (1978). *Family Therapy in Clinical Perspective.* New York, NY: Jason Aronson.

Epston, D. (1994). Extending the conversation. *Family Therapy Networker,* 18, 30-37, 62-63.

Gergen, K.J. (1991). *The Saturated Self: Dilemmas of Identity in Contemporary Life.* New York, NY: Basic Books.

Gergen, K.J. & Gergen, M. (1983). Narratives of the self. In R. Sarbin & K.E. Scheibe (Eds.), *Studies in Social Identity* (pp. 254-273). New York: Praeger.

Gladdings, S.T. (2007). *Family Therapy: History, Theory and Practice.* Upper Saddle River, NJ: Prentice Hall.

Heitler, S.M. (1993). *From Conflict to Resolution: Skills and Strategies for Individual, Couple and Family Therapy.* New York, NY: W.W. Norton and company, Inc.

Hoffman, L. (2002). *Family Therapy: An Intimate History.* New York, NY: W.W. Norton.

Horton, S.L. & Andonian, J.M. (2005). Family as anthology: Towards a metaphoric conceptualization. *The American Journal of Family Therapy,* 33, 85-95.

Hurvitz, N. & Straus, R.A. (1991). *Marriage and Family Therapy: A Sociocognitive Approach.* New York, NY: The Haworth press.

Kallen, J. (2004). Working with chronically ill clients, *Journal of Marital and Family Therapy,* 19, 154-168.

Kurtz, P.D., & Tandy, C.C. (1995). Narrative family interventions. In A.C. Kilpatrick & T.P. Holland (Eds.), *Working with Families* (pp. 177-197). Boston, MA: Allyn & Bacon.

Laird, J. (1991). Women and stories: Restorying women's self constructions. In M. McGoldrick, C. Anderson, & F. Walsh (Eds.), *Women in Families: A Framework for Family Therapy* (pp. 427-450). New York, NY: W.W. Norton & Co.

Miller, I.W. & Keitner, G.I. (1996). Combined medication and psychotherapy in the treatment of chronic mood disorders. *Psychiatric Clinics of North America,* 19, 151-171.

Mills, C.W. (1940). Situated actions and the vocabulary of motives. *American Sociological Review*, 6, 904-913.

Nichols, M.P. & Schwartz, R.C. (2007). *The Essentials of Family Therapy*. Boston, MA: Allyn & Bacon.

Nichols, M.P. & Schwartz, R.C. (2006). *Family Therapy: Concepts and Methods*. Boston, MA: Allyn & Bacon.

Ponzetti, J.J., Jr. (2005). Family beginnings: A comparison of spouses' recollection of courtship. *The Family Journal: Counseling and Therapy for Couples and Families*, 13, 132-138.

Rolland, J.S. (2005). Chronic illness and the family life cycle. In B. Carter & M. McGoldrick (Eds.), *Expanded Family Life Cycle* (pp. 492-511). Boston, MA: Allyn & Bacon.

Stone, E. (1988). *Black Sheep and Kissing Cousins*. New York, NY: Penguin Books.

Vetere, A. (1994). Comment on Wood. *Journal of Family Therapy*, 16, 73-78.

White, M. (1986). Negative explanation, restraint, and double description: A template for family therapy. *Family Process*, 25, 169-184.

White, M. (1989). *Selected Papers*. Adelaide South Australia: Dulwich Centre.

White, M. (1992). Deconstruction and therapy. In M. White & D. Epston (Eds.), *Experience, Contradiction, Narrative, and Imagination* (pp. 109-151). Adelaide South Australia: Dulwich Centre.

White, M. (1993). The histories of the present. In S. Gilligan (Ed.), *Therapeutic Conversations* (pp. 99-121). New York, NY: Norton.

White, M. (1995). *Re-Authoring Lives*. Adelaide, South Australia: Dulwich Centre.

White, M. & Epston, D. (1991). *Narrative Means to Therapeutic Ends*. New York, NY: W.W. Norton.

2

Chronic Illness and the Family Meaning System

Joan D. Atwood
Estelle Weinstein

Abstract

Recently, there has been an increased recognition of the importance of addressing the therapy needs of couples and families where there is a chronically-ill member, signaling the need for couple and family-oriented approaches to address the complex needs of couples and families coping with chronic illness. Chronic illness refers to a chronic, progressive, and degenerative disease. It is the purpose of this chapter to address some of the issues and problems that couples and families with a chronically-ill member may experience, taking life cycle issues into consideration. A distinction is made between the illness experience and the illness behavior. To this we add, the illness meaning, the social and psychological definitions given to the illness and the resultant scripts taken by the ill member, the couple, and by other family members. Implications for therapy are considered throughout.

Pope and Tarlov (1991), based on the National Health Interview Survey (1988), estimate that 33.1 million people have some degree of activity limiting due to chronic illness. Chronic illness refers to a chronic, progressive, and degenerative disease (Devins & Seland, 1987). In the past decade, since the publication of *Family Systems Medicine* in 1982, there has been an increased recognition of the importance of addressing the therapy needs of medical patients and their families within the context of a biopsychosocial model. Major research studies have focused on such chronic illnesses as diabetes, heart disease, and cancer (Krukofsky, 1988) and their effect on the individual; however, the couple and other family members' therapy needs have not received comparable attention.

Minden and Schiffer (1990) emphasize that treatment of chronic illness-related affective disorders is the most neglected area of research, in spite of both the seriousness and the prevalence of emotional disturbances among patients and their families with chronic illness. Although there is a suggested relationship between emotional stress and chronic illness episodes and their prognosis (Warren, Warren, & Cockerill, 1991) and while numerous studies of adjustment factors and the emotional impact of chronic illness allude to the importance of mutually supportive marital relationships (Bezkor & Canedo, 1987; Devins & Seland, 1987; McIvor, Riklan, & Reznikoff, 1984; Ventimiglia, 1986; Zeldow & Pavlou, 1984), there is a significant lack of systemically-oriented couple and family therapy research, which addresses the needs of couples and families where there is a chronically-ill person. Rodgers and Calder (1990) highlight the importance of marital adjustment as a critical factor influencing emotional adjustment to couple relating when there is a chronically-ill member. Minden and Moes (1990) suggest that referral of chronically-ill patients and their families to psychiatrists, psychologists, social workers, marriage and family therapists, or psychiatric nurses "can be helpful to patients with adjustment difficulties and marital and family dysfunction" (p.236). There is an obvious need for more systemically-oriented therapy research to address the complex needs of couples and families coping with chronic illness.

It is the purpose of this chapter to address some of the issues and problems that couples and families with a chronically-ill member may experience, taking life cycle issues into consideration. As suggested by Wynne, Shields & Sirkin (1992), a distinction is made between the "... illness *experience*, the distress, suffering, and perceived loss of well-being, and illness *behavior*, the impaired functioning that is observed by others and is attributed to illness" (p. 5). To this we add, illness *meaning*, the social and psychological definitions given to the illness and the resultant scripts taken on by the family members. Implications for therapy are considered throughout.

Chronic illness is not simply an individual subjective experience; it is interpersonal and social. The definition or meaning an individual gives to an illness is profoundly influenced by and influences that person's social world. The social culture and the social networks shape and are shaped by the individual's experiences. The meaning of the illness is shared and negotiated in everyday interactions and it is deeply embedded in the social world. As such it is inseparable from the structure and processes that constituted that social world (Atwood, 1996). Thus, to explore the definitional processes involved in chronic illness is to explore the individual's interpersonal relations and the resultant meaning system.

Unexpected, health-related life events raise many questions for therapists and other health service providers. What are the factors that determine the onset of serious, chronic, and degenerative diseases and how does the progression of an illness affect families? To what extent does gender, the life cycle stage of the players at the onset of the illness (childhood/adulthood), roles, couple relationships, social support systems, and finances contribute to the way families cope. Can family systems be strengthened rather than weakened in the face of health problems? How do marital and family dynamics, belief systems, rules, and boundaries determine the physical well-being of its members and their ability to adapt to physical health problems? This article provides a foundation for understanding the role illness plays in family systems and the implications for effective intervention.

A Bio-Psycho-Social Perspective

Until recently, disease was thought to be a function of the breakdown of bio-physiological processes (Engel, 1980a; Serafino, 1990). This bio-medical model of disease assumed that there were distinct separations between the mind and the body. Within this framework, health was an exclusive function of a person's physical state. While there are some changes emerging, the medical system in this country is still primarily a product of this model (Serafino, 1990), and within this belief system, interventions consist almost entirely of medical technologies. The medical system concerns itself with the treatment of the biology of an illness in an individual. Little clinical attention is paid to the person's mental health and even less attention is paid to his or her family.

Only recently in our history have we begun to consider a newer, theoretical conceptualization of health and disease known as the biopsychosocial model (Engel, 1977; Engel, 1980b). This multi-factored perspective suggests that an interaction of the biological, psychological, and social aspects of a person's life are the determinants of his or her health, the onset of illness, and often the prognosis. Even the immune system, which was thought to be a strictly biological response, is now thought to be influenced by emotional factors, and even the course of chronic illness is now considered largely determined by lifestyle behaviors (Sarafino, 1990). Now, it is believed that psychological factors, such as cognition, emotion, and motivation for behavior and mental processes contribute to a person's proneness for illness and also to the person's speed of recovery (i.e., positive attitudes decrease recovery time, negative attitudes extend recovery time) (Sarafino, 1990). Thus, the social systems in which a person functions (family, work, and community) influences their belief systems, lifestyle, and experiences with health and how ultimately they use health providers. These recursively interact with many other health determining factors.

Out of this broader bio-psycho-social model has come evidence of changes in the preparation of medical providers and changes in the thinking of mental health personnel, especially in the field of marriage and family therapy, where the specialty, family systems medicine, has emerged. This thinking offers an opportunity for medical practitioners and family therapists to collaborate in their efforts to help families with serious, chronic, and debilitating illnesses. Such collaboration means learning about the training, theoretical paradigms, languages, and working styles of each profession. This serves to decrease power issues and increase communication between them (McDaniel, 1992). For family therapists, it means understanding the biology of disease and the medical approaches to treatment. For the medical practitioner, it means learning about how family systems affect health and how health status affects families. For the family, it means that there will be a respectful acknowledgment of the disruptions and emotional responses that an illness may inflict upon a family. This approach focuses on the family's strengths and supports.

Utilizing family social workers and family therapists for organizing family conferences between the chronically-ill family member, the other family members, and the primary care physician can be of great value. In addition, these mental health professionals can play a key role in coordinating medical and mental health services for the family coping with chronic illness by educating the family about community resources such as support groups, etc.

Family Life Cycle Considerations

Biopsychosocial factors change systematically in response to developmental stages (Sarafino, 1990). For example, the biological functioning of older people is challenged by many more chronic diseases than middle-aged people or children, just by virtue of more lengthy normal wear and tear on their bodies. Rolland (1989) proposes a model, which emphasizes the intertwining of evolutionary threads: the illness and the individual family life cycles (p.433). He proposes a typology which conceptualizes distinctions of (1) onset, (2) course, (3) outcome, and (4) degree of incapacitation. By combining the kinds of onset (acute versus chronic), course (progressive versus constant versus relapsing/ episodic), outcome (fatal versus shortened life span versus nonfatal) and incapacitation (present versus absent) into a grid format, Rolland generates a typology of thirty-two potential psychosocial types of illness (p. 438). In addition to the core themes, he also utilizes the context of three major disease phases: (1) crisis, (2) chronic, and (3) terminal, in order to follow the history of the disease process. This facilitates an appreciation and understanding for the ever-changing needs and requirements of the patient, the couple, and the family system over the course of the family life cycle. In addition, he (p. 447) incorporates the concepts of centrifugal (forces that push members apart) versus centripetal (forces that push members together) family styles and phases in the family life cycle (Beavers, 1982; Beavers & Voeller, 1983) as a means of integrating family, individual, and illness development.

It is particularly useful to bear in mind the significant centripetal pull, which chronic disease exerts on a multigenerational family system, and its potential impact on the couple's boundaries and the established hierarchy within the family. For example, if the couple has children, the therapist's interest in their adjustment process may prompt a sharing of the parents' concerns and a discussion of problem-solving options. This may also have the effect of strengthening the parental hierarchy. For couples who wish to have children, there may be concerns regarding genetic factors relating to the chronic illness and the potential risks of pregnancy.

Life Event

Becoming chronically ill is a life event. A life event may be broadly described as an array of experiences that require significant changes in the ongoing life pattern of the individual (Holmes & Masuda, 1974). Life events may be categorized in three ways: normative age-graded events, such as marriage, childbirth, or menopause; normative history-graded events, such as wars, economic depressions, etc.; and non-normative events, such as illness, disability or job loss. Chronic illness falls into the last category and as such necessitates a redefinitional process by all family members. This redefinitional process involves the incorporation of the idea that a family member is ill. This is a continual, co-emergent process, which is played out by different family members in different ways. It primarily involves a construction of a reality centered around the concepts of sickness and disease, often involving isolation and control. The "sick" family member becomes more isolated as those who are healthy take on more controlling attributes. The process is painful, not deliberate, yet generally involves the taking in of the symptomatic patient definition.

Life events may be understood broadly as experiences that require "significant change in the ongoing life pattern of the individual" (Holmes & Masuda, 1974, p.46). Hultsch & Deutsch (1981) classified events in three categories. The first, normative age-graded events, are determined largely by biological capacity or social norms; and accordingly, their timing and duration are similar for many people. Representative examples include marriage, childbirth, menopause, and retirement. The second category, normative history-graded events, are experienced by most members of a cohort. Representative samples are wars, political shifts, economic depressions, and mass immigrations. The third category consists of non-normative events. These are weakly correlated with life stage or historical time, which are idiosyncratic in occurrence, and limited to a small proportion of the population. Examples include illness, disability, and job loss.

The sociological impact of family or cultural membership affects belief systems, family rituals, and the different ways people use the healthcare system at different times during the life cycle. The response to a child's illness, the role sick family members play, the respect for or willingness to use health professionals—all have roots in family of origin dynamics. Hence, interventions that increase people's ability to delay the onset of or cope with serious illness must include an understanding of disease entities, expected physical prognoses, and psycho-social implications, especially interpersonal relationships, coping styles, and present and past family dynamics. When the onset of chronic illness coincides with transitional points in the individual or family life cycle, there is perhaps an even greater risk of problems. "The added centripetal pull exerted by a progressive disease increases the risk of reversing normal family disengagement (i.e., child going away to college) freezing a family into a permanent state of fusion" (Rolland, 1989, p. 450). An important aspect of therapy with couples in the reversal of such centripetal overreactions involves frank discussions of what they see as realistic alternatives and options.

The Social Construction of Illness

As stated earlier, much of the writings on chronic illness sees disease through a bio-medical lens meaning that chronic illness is looked at primarily as an organic phenomenon characterized by gradual deterioration, occurring to an individual, and currently having no cure. Chronic illness is diagnosed using biomedical assessment techniques and the care of the individual is under medical authority, which may involve the prescription of medication and/or hospitalization. However, seeing chronic illness only through a biomedical lens is limiting in that it gives little consideration to the social factors affecting disease definition, experience, and/or progression, including the balance of power in the relationship of caregiver and patient. Using only bio-medical lenses to view the chronically ill results in the medicalization of the disease, the individual, and the family, which could lead to a justification of control "for the good of the patient."

Berger and Luckmann (1966) describe social construction assumptions, which question the above medical model approach. They describe social constructions as the consensual recognition of the coherence or realness of a constructed reality, plus the socialization process by which people acquire this reality. The social constructionist approach believes that all humans participate in social action and interaction, which takes place in a sociocultural environment. This sociocultural environment includes "taken for granted" assumptions, rules, and beliefs about what it means to be sick, to have a disease, etc. It is within this framework of shared definitions that patients and caregivers interact and behave accordingly. And it is this social context that determines individuals' scripts for behavior.

Scripts are plans that people have about what they are doing and what they are going to do. They justify situations that are in agreement with them and challenge those that are not. They constitute the available repertoire of socially-recognized acts and statuses, and roles and the rules governing them. Scripts operate at a social, personal and intrapsychic level (Atwood, 1992). Within this framework, shared knowledge of chronic illness is a collective definition, part of the sociocultural world of the person with that of their caregivers.

The social constructionist model acknowledges that a problem or belief about an illness is a construct of both the family and the therapist and not simply a function of the sick individual's situation. It recognizes both the family and the therapist's beliefs about how the illness influences the way the family organizes around the illness. It focuses on the therapist respectfully identifying the family's beliefs about what the illness is, how the illness affects their family, and what changes the family would like to have in their response to the illness. The family's perceptions and beliefs change about the illness experience and the family is able to utilize alternative responses to help alleviate pain, suffering, or restrictions.

Narrative Focus

More recently, there has been a recognition that language plays a crucial role in how people "see" and thus experience illness. According to this narrative line of inquiry in the social and behavioral sciences, people revise accounts of life experience in the face of unexpected or adverse events so as to maintain a sense of coherence, continuity and meaning (Gergen & Gergen, 1983). In this sense narrative processes can be understood as reflexive efforts to cope with negative life outcomes and to deal with the impact of change and loss. In spite of definitional problems inherent in the concept (Sarbin, 1986), theoreticians concur that narratives must organize events in such a way that they demonstrate a sense of coherence as well as a sense of direction or movement over time (Bruner, 1990; Mishler, 1986; Ricoer, 1981). The assumption is that narratives carry implications for the well-being of the narrators and point to a range of potential outcomes. In so doing, they reflect a valuative condition and provide an indication of events to come.

In effect, this suggests that each person becomes a historian of the self, developing an internally-consistent interpretation of the life cycle so that past, present, and future are experienced as congruent. The assumption is that such processes work to preserve a sense of coherence and continuity in identity and self, which are seen as critical determinants of mental health (Antonovsky, 1987; Basch, 1976; Cohler, 1982; Erikson, 1963; Kohut, 1977). Here the therapist can assist the family in mourning the loss of their pre-illness expectations, discovering their resources and defining new meanings for themselves. By obtaining information about the illness and learning about other families' experiences, the family can normalize what is happening to them while taking control of what may seem to be an uncontrollable situation. It is important that the ill member actively participate in creating the narrative, collecting information, and restructuring family responsibilities.

Research about Illness

It is important to note that a good deal of the research that addresses the interaction between family and health is anecdotal and lacks solid design, thereby compromising our ability to generalize the results. The literature that does exist primarily addresses medical conditions and the burdens associated with the provision of care (by spouse or other) often to the exclusion of how the interpersonal relationships in the family are affected or affect the physical health of its members (Creasey, 1990).

Hence, interrelationships between social and psychological factors, including economic and demographic variables and their influence on the impact of illnesses and family dynamics, has largely been ignored. What is presented below is a discussion that defines terminology and provides a framework for understanding the important issues with regard to chronic, serious illness and the family.

Until recently, the medical and scientific community had virtually conquered or controlled most communicable diseases (e.g., smallpox, measles, diphtheria, etc.). Even in the sphere of the Human Immunodeficiency Virus (HIV), the major causes of death in this country became chronic degenerative diseases especially heart disease, cancer and stroke. While HIV infection is communicable, it destroys the immune system and persons with Acquired Immune Deficiency Syndrome (AIDS) actually die of opportunistic chronic diseases.

Chronic diseases are those that develop over time, progress symptomatically, result in permanent, compromising changes in the person's health, are mediated by lifestyle, and often have a genetic component. The effects of a chronic disease, while in some cases are predictable, more often vary over time from patient to patient. On the other hand, serious communicable or infectious diseases that also affect health status are transmissible from one person to another and have a limited time recovery or ultimately result in more chronic conditions if they do not end in a relatively swift death.

While risk factors for chronic diseases have historically been identified as behavioral or genetic in the diagnosed person, recently health professionals have begun to explore interpersonal relationship factors as they relate to risk for illness. Some of the questions considered are: To what extent does personality, lifestyle, behaviors, etc. in one spouse increase the likelihood of serious illness in the other? Can characteristics in a well spouse be the cause of an illness in the partner? How will individual characteristics or couple dynamics affect the way a couple lives with an illness when it occurs? How do parental characteristics affect children's experiences with illness and their belief systems?

Haynes (1983) was one of the first to demonstrate less conventional risks for coronary heart disease (CHD), including those associated with and heightened by certain characteristics in a spouse. Swan, Carmelli, & Roseman (1986) studying this phenomenon named it "cross-spouse" risk factors" (p. 172). They found that such factors, such as higher social mobility, increased life pessimism, high school or above education, higher levels of activity and dominance, were significantly important to women married to men with CHD who were also Type A personalities. While these characteristics are significantly present in their spouses, what has not yet been determined is if, and how, this notion of interactive causality functions. Had the disease in the husbands resulted in the wife's pessimism, which in turn affected his coping or, is her increased activity or dominance a response to his illness?

Levenson and Gottman (in Swan & Carmelli...) studying marital interaction and satisfaction as they relate to serious illness found greater physiological symptomatology among couples who reported dissatisfaction with and conflict in their marriages than with those who reported being satisfied. A serious illness often results in the disruption in the social and recreational activities for the diagnosed person as well as the other family members; but, it also has specific implications for a marital couple. Research indicates that an ill person's contact with friends outside the family usually diminishes considerably because of such things as; medical limitations, physical exhaustion, and embarrassment about physical appearance that has resulted from the illness. This in turn limits the spouse's social activities. For example, in the case where an insulin-dependent diabetic needs to adhere to a strict diet, attending dinners and parties might be too tempting. Or, in the case of a cancer patient undergoing chemotherapy or radiation treatment, the ill person may be just too exhausted to be sociable. If there is disfigurement resulting from an illness, the person may be afraid of rejection from close friends or people staring at him or her in public places. Thus, the couple may avoid these social functions. The spouse or other family members may begin to feel isolated, in need of social stimulation, guilty if they partake and often angry at the ill spouse. Swan (1986) found that for up to a year or so after a diagnosis or onset of a serious illness, spouses of an ill partner reported increased depression, anxiety, and a major disruption in their routine. Yet, over time the couple's balance appeared to return.

In addition to the emotional distress that occurs in an ill spouse, the well spouse often experiences a revisit of, or a host of new physical and psychological symptoms of their own. And, the data indicate that well spouse difficulties significantly influence the coping and psychological well-being of the ill partner (Manne & Zautra, 1989). This research explains that when a relationship is stable and positive, couples are better able to withstand the struggle of serious illness and in some cases report their relationship is even strengthened by it; whereas, if the relationship is troubled it may be destroyed (Shlain, 1979). Mullan (1983) looked at longer term effects (over ten years after a coronary incident), and found that less than 20% reported less satisfaction with their marriage and 25% actually reported increased satisfaction after chronic illness entered the family. While the passage of time generally helps people adjust to new and possibly life-threatening life cycle situations, some couples report that their relationships and commitment deepened as they reevaluated what was important to them.

Reactions to a Diagnosis of a Serious Illness

A diagnosis of a serious illness provides medical practitioners with a label and frame of reference with which to approach patients. While the diagnosis speaks to bio-physiological factors, it does not begin to suggest the psycho-social demands that the diagnosed individual, couple, and family may face (Rolland, 1993). The label of the disease itself often addresses the beliefs and past experiences of the people involved with the illness. When a person is diagnosed with cancer, for example, several expectations may be made. If there is the belief that cancer is not "treatable" or "beatable," and is physiologically devastating, then, compensations often begin even before any severe symptoms manifest themselves. The person may develop a "sick" role by virtue of the diagnosis alone. Here people tend to surrender their responsibilities to others. This can result in a shift in the family power and further encourages the diagnosed person to define him or herself as no longer capable. This sick role may have some advantages, for example, in a disease that runs a particular course it may give the diagnosed person an opportunity to rest and recover with a respite from the usual responsibilities. On the other hand, it may discourage the person from maximizing their coping abilities. Even in the case where the disease requires the ill person's constant self-monitoring, people who have taken on the sick role tend to relinquish their decision-making rights and caretaking to health providers or significant others. On the other hand, some people may believe that cancer is not a death sentence, but an opportunity to deepen their lives, to bring new meanings to their relationships, to increase their religious affiliations or to take control and "be strong," perhaps for the first time in their lives. As a result, these responses can result in many positive changes in family systems.

Shontz (1975) outlines a common sequence of reactions persons tend to have when they are diagnosed with a serious illness. The first reaction, shock, is characterized by bewilderment. The person behaves in an automatic fashion, exhibiting feelings of detachment from the immediate situation. These avoidance reactions are a means of getting distance from the overwhelming feelings. In the second phase a person may exhibit disorganized thinking, and feelings of loss, grief, and despair. This is more typical when a diagnosis comes without warning to a seemingly healthy person. The third phase is characterized by a denial of the circumstances, along with an acknowledgment of the existence of the health problem. However, in most cases, the reality of the situation returns slowly as the person's ability to cope increases. If avoidance and denial are maintained over too long a period of time, a person may become immobilized, especially in his or her ability to gather information about the problem. This can prohibit them from making timely decisions about their treatment or care needs. This could also result in another family member taking over the decision-making role, evaluating treatment options, and providing daily care. It is in this situation that power shifts, role reversals and conflicting triangulations occur. Or, as the family surrounds the ill member, it can result in bonding more closely, strengthening each member into a support system. These increases in family bonding and support also may increase healing and promote coping. While shock is a fairly consistent initial response (Shontz, 1975), some persons who become ill do not become disorganized or evidence avoidance behaviors. They seem much more in control and accepting of the illness and begin to structure their lives around the necessary accommodations.

It is family of origin tapes, sociocultural beliefs about illness and economic and social circumstances that effect these more immediate reactions to serious health problems. Peoples' beliefs about the identity of an illness (Meyerowitz, 1983), the cause, the duration, and the consequences of their conditions are important predictors of their ability to adjust.

Health Locus of Control

Reactions to health concerns have also been explained by theories of "locus of control" and self-efficacy (Phares, 1987). Rotter (1966), developed the original scales for measuring internal and external locus of control, and Wallston, Wallston, & DeVellis (1978) applied these concepts to a health-related measure called the Multidimensional Health Locus of Control Scales. People with an "internal locus of control" believe that they are in control of their own successes and failures. Hence, people with a powerful internal locus of control believe that something they do or do not do determines their health status. These individuals are also more likely to think that their ability to overcome a serious illness is determined by themselves and their behaviors. They verbalize things like, "If I give in to this, I will get sicker," or "I'll decide what is best for me!" They also tend to make their own informed decisions about their care and adhere to regimens that they believe will work.

People with an external "powerful other" locus of control are more likely to believe that professionals or others outside themselves determine their illness successes or failures. These individuals believe that the outcome of their illness is determined by their doctor or surgeon and generally leave their care in the hands of a medical professional, basically doing only what they are told.

Chance locus of control is exhibited by people who believe that luck, fate, or God determines their successes and failures. Persons with a chance locus of control will say things like, "If I'm lucky, I'll get over this" or "If my time is up, it's up, and nothing I can do can change that." As people move from middle to older age, their notions of chance or powerful other locus of control tends to increase and they are more likely to turn to medical professionals to make their health-related decisions (Lachman, 1986). People who optimize their health by living healthy lifestyles believe that they can determine their own health status. People who exhibit less stress and those who tend to cope with serious illnesses tend to have stronger internal loci of control.

Eternality or internality of control also influences the way people use the healthcare system. Individuals who hold belief systems that incorporate notions like "the doctor knows best" and turn their care over to the practitioner are less likely to seek second medical opinions and medical procedures unless their primary physician suggests it. Few questions are asked about the treatment process, treatment expectations, or the protocol and they tend to perform as the "good patient." On the other hand, believing in fate or God often causes people not to seek treatment or can limit the treatment they seek because they do not believe it will make any difference in the outcome.

As stated before, belief in one's ability to control health-related events and where a person falls on the locus of control continuum is largely determined by family of origin experiences, culture, and social groups. In the case of couples who hold diverse beliefs about their ability to control or determine outcomes, when a chronic illness diagnosis is made, a more chaotic response is generally observed.

Poor physical health in general and especially chronic disease tends to erode individuals' sense of control over their life and destiny (Baltes, 1990). Emotional well-being is likely to decline as health status is severely compromised. Hence, the tasks for managing serious chronic illnesses include achieving some measure of control over the symptoms of the illness, adhering to complex treatment regimens, coping with the uncertainty of a prognosis, supporting and maintaining family, work, social relationships, and other usual responsibilities within the parameters of the illness, and continuing to set goals and plans for the future. Furthermore, a sense of self-efficacy or the belief that, "We can succeed at something we want to do," is another factor in maintaining a sense of control in the face of serious illness (Bandura, 1977) .

Adherence/Compliance

When a crisis period of serious illness subsides, the medical treatment plan for controlling the disease and preventing additional problems is to a major extent reliant upon the ability of a person to select and adhere to medical protocols that have been found to be successful. It is important for the family to support these protocols. This is presently referred to as "adherence" (DiMatteo, 1982; Turk, 1991). In the medical literature, adherence occurs at two levels: (1) primary adherence, which refers to a person's ability or willingness to carry out activities that prevent the initial onset of illness, and (2) secondary and tertiary adherence, which refers to following prescribed procedures that are aimed at controlling a specific health condition from getting worse (Turk, 1991). The terminology "compliance," rather than adherence was more commonly used in the past, suggesting that people with diseases follow the steps assigned to them by medical practitioners. The present notion of "adherence" requires that people make informed decisions, by selecting and then adhering to a specific protocol. It is this commitment to the decision and the following of the particular protocol that is believed to determine the physical outcome of an illness rather than the medical effectiveness of a particular drug or procedure (Epstein, 1984). This taking of action on one's own behalf often results in feelings of self-confidence, an increased sense of well-being, and an increased likelihood of participating in ancillary healthful behaviors that ultimately limit or control the effects of serious illness. Movement from the terminology "compliance" to "adherence" in the health field indicates shared decision-making about health behaviors between practitioners and patients.

Several factors have been identified as affecting people's ability to adhere to specific health behaviors. These include: a simplified understanding of the protocol or regimen; an ability to implement a protocol with a minimum of life changes; satisfaction with and a feeling of confidence in the source of the regimen; the specificity of the regimen including such factors as length of time needed, cost, etc.; and the social and psychological factors in the person's environment that influence the activities (Sarafino, 1990; Turk, 1991). When individuals make a commitment to a protocol that is in concert with their belief systems and the roles and behaviors of their significant others, there is a greater likelihood that the process will be followed. Sometimes, individuals have a person in their family that they look to for family's health matters and decisions. Adherence successes can be closely associated with approval from this pseudo family doctor.

Often, the family's support in adherence activities deepens the family's trust and intimacy; however, families have been known to sabotage the process. In the author's clinical practice, it was suggested to a man who recently suffered a heart attack that diet and exercise would help him to control his disease and decrease his risk of sudden death. He discussed with his wife what this would mean to each of them. The family ate together often and their dietary habits did not resemble the required diet. Moreover, the only social activities the couple participated in together were during dinners out. At first the adjustments seemed easy as the risk of dying from heart disease was central to their fears. The family shopping and meal preparing was done by the wife and she indicated her complete support of the new eating behavior and the healthier eating habits by decreasing her own weight. The exercise protocol required him to exercise regularly at a rehabilitation center after work which, while she completely supported it, would decrease their dinner time together. As distance from the acute heart attack and the possibility of death was achieved over time, the couple began to lose interest in maintaining the healthier behaviors. The restrictions it posed on their social structure became problematic for them. As his health became less central to their fears, she began to pay less attention to what they ate and he went back to his "couch potato" evenings. They argued frequently, she accusing him of not taking care of himself and leaving all of the burden to her and he accusing her of putting him at risk for another heart attack by planning social dinners with friends at places where he could not choose healthy meals. At a support group they met other couples with serious CHD illnesses who encouraged them to join a local health club and a bicycle traveling group. The definition of themselves as a "diseased couple" receded as these new social activities enabled them to participate in a new, healthier social life, assisting them to create renewed interest in each other.

Implications for The Family

Individuals and their families deal with a wide range of issues when a chronic illness enters the family. Issues can range from existing issues prior to the illness, to fear of abandonment, fear of death, spiritual beliefs, and exhaustion from caretaking and interaction with the medical community (Atwood & Ruiz, 1992; Harrington & Messer, 1994; McDaniel, Hepworth, & Doherty, 1993; Rolland, 1994).

Although a serious illness manifests itself in one member of the family, it is perceived as an intruder by other family members. Eventually the illness itself becomes an independent functioning member of the system, with its own separate identity. It is demanding in that it requires readjustment of schedules, roles, finances, etc. It elicits anger in that it is often uncontrollable and causes pain and fear. It is selfish in that it must be attended to whenever it demands, despite other activities or interests. It is isolating in that it often changes intimacy and friendship patterns.

While the family's task is to meet the ill person's medical and other caregiving needs, the emotional well-being of the entire system is challenged. This may lead to couple or family discord that continues to decrease health status, which in turn negatively affects family dynamics.

Family scripts and experiences with illness have implications to the functioning of the system and its ability to adapt. If, for example, the family has a definitional system, which includes ideas that the illness could have been prevented or that it was caused by themselves or another family member, then a place for blame is sought, i.e., the family diet was not healthy because it was not a priority of the meal preparer, or the ill person worked too many hours on his/her job, or the children caused "too much stress." These types of thought process attempt to explain or offer some level of control over what feels like an uncontrollable situation. Hostility, low self-esteem, and other negative patterns may develop as the family system is threatened. These patterns tend to create distance from the problem or create distance between family members, often closing down communication and leaving little room for accommodation to the new situation. In some cases, blame is sought outside the family system. Here, it is usually directed toward the medical profession, i.e., the doctor incorrectly diagnosed the ailment or took too long to recognize it. In these cases there is a loss in faith in the medical system, which may result in the delay of necessary treatment.

The demands of an illness often deplete energy, dissolve optimism, and create depression. If the chronically-ill person experiences depression, it may lead to other family members having increased risk for depression themselves (Coyne, 1986). Also, those family systems with existing problems tend to adjust less well to their new situation and exaggeration of the negative patterns may occur (Swan, Carmelli, & Rosenman, 1986).

When an illness compromises the diagnosed member's physical capabilities and personality characteristics, there is a constant struggle on the part of the person to maintain equilibrium. In some cases, this struggle creates growth, development, new closeness, and trust in the primary or family relationships as needed shifts in roles, power, and responsibilities emerge. However, in other cases, as the person's self care capabilities decrease, resentment, jealousy, and/or feelings of overburdenedness may occur as the family relationships deteriorate. The task of maintaining the family support and intimacy is ongoing for all members. In order to effectively accommodate and regain equilibrium, it is helpful for family members challenged by serious illness to receive information about the expected patterns of the particular disorder or illness and the resultant practical and emotional demands these patterns may create for them over time (Rolland, 1993). In addition, it is helpful for them to address their mythical notions about the illness in light of the medical realities about the health problem, and to "language" their fears with each other. Open communication for all family members is crucial. Living with secrets can encourage fear and guilt. Since all family members may be anticipating loss, it is helpful to discuss the issues of health care, living wills, powers of attorney and finances in the present. This may help the family to keep their affairs in order at a time when they are under tremendous stress.

The onset of an illness, whether an acute attack or a gradual development of symptoms, has implications for how families will function, as does the nature of the expected progression of a particular disease (progressive, constant or relapsing) and the expected outcome for survival. Can a course of events be outlined for an individual upon diagnosis, including the degree of disability and pain that is likely to occur or is the future vague and uncertain (Rolland, 1993)? What medical interventions are available and how can people access them?

The family's definition of health and illness and the meaning they give it contributes to their ability to set boundaries around a health problem. Finding the appropriate place for the illness so that it does not become the central focus of the family serves to limit the boundaries of the disease. When boundaries are not established and maintained, the illness invades all aspects of the family system and the family becomes uni-focused. The individual's physical limitations become the family's limitations. Here,

plans and activities for all members center around the activities associated with the illness (going to doctors, taking medication, etc.). In this
case, the therapist can commend the family and individual's strengths.
S/he can offer information, validate and normalize emotional responses,
draw forth family support, encourage respite, and reinforce the continu-
ance of family rituals. It is important for the therapist to assist the family
in dealing with those problems that the family have collaborated and
contracted to change. Any interventions should match the family's style
of relating, and interventions should be linked to the family's strengths
and previous useful solution strategies.

Enmeshment/Disengagement

Disengagement may occur among family members who cannot cope
or are unable to caregive in ways that are acceptable to themselves or the
system. Others may become so enmeshed in the symptoms and disease
entity that it becomes difficult to distinguish between the sick member
and the others who are well. While the ill person is still able to maintain
his or her past roles or tasks with some modifications, the enmeshed
family might usurp that ability and elicit a lack of competence. When the
sick role becomes assigned to an individual with a previously dependent
spouse, that spouse when encouraged may become stronger and better
functioning. But, as they do so, there is an obvious shift in the power in
the relationship away from the ill spouse.

Inverted Hierarchies

Family structure involves system boundaries, roles, sanctions, attitudes, and values that guide family members. Thus, it is these structures
that are challenged by the introduction of chronic illness into the family
system. Timing is also an important component of the systems well-
being. In some cases the type of serious illness determines the timing
factor. In cases where the onset of an illness is acute, changes tend to
occur very quickly. Often the ill person is hospitalized during acute
attacks. In an acute phase of illness, the family may become off balance as much of the decision making falls to the medical community
and the major family tasks become survival and treatment. Family
members spend much of their time at the hospital. The outside world
and the day-to-day activities recede as the illness takes the foreground
again. Social relationships may change as family members become
unavailable to their friends, especially when they are involved in the
immediacy of the illness.

When a person enters a hospital or other medical in-patient facility, the family's identity is lost as is the ill person's. The rules and behaviors specific to that family are disregarded as the hospital rules become the governing forces. The concerns of the hospital staff center on the "patient" in need of services rather than on the individual with an independent identity or a person as a member of a family system. The care and day-to-day life become routinized according to hospital schedules. The ill person may take on the role of the "good patient," giving over their destiny to the medical staff. This medical environment is conducive to doctors/nurses and patients creating parent-child relationships or inverted hierarchies. The non-assertive family often is carried along with this redefinition, feeling safe that someone in authority has taken over the caretaking.

The Rigid Hierarchy

In other situations, patients and their families fight hard not to give up their rights and roles to the hospital facility and the personnel. The complication of maintaining one's independence and needing to be cared for is a difficult balance. Family members often rebel against the routine and the limited access they have, not only to each other but to information about care. Anger is not an uncommon emotion.

Triangulations

In some cases, a more chronic debilitating illness results after the acute phase. In these situations, medical personnel may become a permanent, important sphere of influence on the family, if not full-fledged members of the system. In some cases the medical practitioner is "triangulated" (refers to the recruitment of a third person into the family system for purposes of lowering the intensity of stress and anxiety and to regain stability) in the family system. The triangulated relationship may be with the caregiver or the patient and can contribute to conflict and confusion in the system.

If the acute phase ends and the person survives, a period of rehabilitation or healing begins. The participants in the system work toward regaining their balance and helping the ill person maximize their resulting health functioning. At this time, what occurs is an assessment and understanding of the more chronic conditions and disabilities that will remain a part of the person's life forever.

The threats of loss and disability have considerable implications to the family's ability to function. Changes in physical appearance and emotional state result in the sick person revisiting most of the important components of their life, roles, and future plans. As a result of the illness, some of these plans may vanish while others may become stronger as a new identity is sought. The family system reorganizes as the chronic illness is given its family position. Changes in the rules that govern the system are effectively made as the family becomes centrally or peripherally (depending upon the severity of the symptoms) organized around the illness. When there is a particular health problem that has an expected progression, the changes tend to be more subtle and can be planned and managed as the family adapts to the definition of the disease. Time allows for adaptations with less disruption to occur as a full understanding of the impending physical changes emerge more slowly.

The Roller Coaster

Chronic illnesses like cancer can have periods of remission between bouts of serious debilitation, which can create a roller coaster type of effect. During remission, there is a slow "lulling" away from the immediacy of loss, fear, and suffering. During the reoccurrence periods, impending loss, helplessness, feelings of anger, confusion, and fear are likely to return. Here the individual's short range goals and future plans are severely disrupted and life seems to take on an unpredictable dimension.

Finances

In situations where an ill spouse holds a primary role like providing for the family's income or child care, there may be fear of the future. In addition, sometimes guilt arises. An ill spouse may have to make decisions that demand acknowledging the outcomes of his or her illness. Here the challenge for the family is to verbalize the emotions and assist the ill person to maintain as much independence as possible while releasing responsibilities. This can sometimes be accomplished by shifting and changing roles rather than giving them up.

Life-Cycle Issues

The lifecycle of the sick person and the developmental stages of the other family members has implications for the family's ability to adapt. The impact of disabilities on the expectations and skill mastery at one stage may differ considerably from another but no matter what the stage of life, illness and disability has a profound affect on family systems. For example, if chronic illness enters the family in a child who has not achieved independent living skills, it has a different impact than if it occurred later in the child's life. If a certain level of success is achieved at a career that requires skills that cannot be maintained, it may have a different effect on the individual and the family than if it occurred at the end of the career or before that particular career had been selected.

Rolland (1993) suggests that families need support in establishing "beliefs that sustain hope and empower, instead of those that foster blame, shame, or guilt" (p.15). Independence and an ability to maintain optimal functioning within the parameters of the illness needs to be fostered. Furthermore, to avoid hostile imbalances in power and control, he identifies the need for families to see health problems as couple or family problems.

Serious chronic illness can create a reconstruction of the past to find meaning for the future. People who have remission from serious illness can achieve a much greater meaning for each life event. From this powerful experience of vulnerability can be opportunity for the strengthening of marital bonds, emotional intimacy, deep expressions of caring and commitment, opening communications and increasing trust (Chekryn, 1984). The disruption in the family that occurs when chronic illness enters the system may contribute to positive changes. Family members can develop new and better ways to interact with one another.

Chronic Illness and Children

Bronchial asthma, juvenile diabetes, leukemia, and other cancers are among the more serious chronic and debilitating diseases that affect children and young adults. While once fatal, as a result of medical technology and effective pharmacology, children often live with these illnesses and their related problems for the whole of their lives.   .

The preconceived notion about a chronic illness has implications for a family's ability to cope and adjust. Marteau & Johnston (1986), in their study of parents with children who have chronic diseases, found that parents rated diseases that their own children had as less serious than those of other children. Moreover, there were less negative feelings about a health problem that they were living with than one that their child did not have. This ability of the family to see others' problems as worse than their own tends to increase their ability to cope.

In early childhood, the parent child relationship can be interfered with by long in-patient separations where the child's needs are met by the doctors or nurses. These have implications in the maintenance of the family hierarchy where there are physical disabilities that may interfere with attempts at independence, children's self-confidence may be compromised. Over-compensating parents may inhibit their child's developmental task mastery or the child can become rebellious in an attempt to push out the boundaries.

The peer system in later childhood and early adolescence provides a yardstick by which children measure themselves and develop their self-image. If a child has a chronic illness at this life cycle stage, peer relationships may become problematic. Peers can be cruel and may make it more difficult for the child to develop a social network, especially if the disabilities are severely restricting. When this happens, the family may overcompensate and become strongly protective of the child, meeting more of the child's needs than necessary. This is a particularly crucial and difficult time for families, as children with chronic illness attempt to negotiate adolescence through close friendships and personal values that are different from their families. Sometimes the withdrawal and loneliness experienced by an ill child results in anger and self-recrimination. If the family has been vested in maintaining the adolescent's health without encouraging their maximum input, adolescent rebellion may be expressed in refusal of treatment or medication.

When the day-to-day activities of a family are adjusted by an ill child's needs, other family members especially other siblings may become angry and resentful at the same time as they experience guilt for any attention they do receive. Wilson-Pessano & McNabb (1989) found that the diagnosed child's care often took away from the needs or restricted the other children in the family. Siblings in a family with an ill child adapted best when schedules, visits, and vacations, were adjusted to the total family's needs wherever possible rather than entirely to the diagnosed child's. When sibling's identities and importance in the family are supported and appreciated, less resentment and anger was felt. Where there is a family's encouragement in maintaining an ill child's involvement in his or her own care and decision making (where developmentally appropriate), the child's confidence and coping ability are maximized.

Shapiro's (1986) research looked at maternal influences on families with chronically-ill children and found that a mother's ability to adjust correlated strongly to overall family adaptation. Where mothers were depressed, siblings and other family members had negative feelings toward the ill child. Moreover, when families are unable to express their frustrations, fears, and angers, the family's ability to accommodate to the changes was weakened. The interactional patterns, communication, and feelings of the entire family unit are important therapeutic material (Minuchin, Rosman & Baker, 1978). The resources external to the family system (i.e., financial, childcare, etc.) can support or weaken the stability of the family and its ability to accommodate to the illness. Helping families with the multitude of support services they might need to survive a serious childhood illness requires a multi-systemic intervention.

Less explored in the literature are the problems young children face when a parent is seriously ill. The separation and the fragility of the diagnosed parent may result in feelings of insecurity in the child. The protective environment of the family seems compromised when attention is placed on the ill parent. Temporary caregivers may not set appropriate boundaries so that children may feel particularly vulnerable. Children may feel excluded from the family interactions especially when they are given little or no explanation for the changes in the system or about their parent's health status. There is more than one case where the parent of a young child was taken to the hospital where s/he died and the child was given no explanation whatsoever, other than "Mommy /Daddy went to heaven." Later in therapy sessions, the adult explores the anger the child may have experienced from feelings of abandonment.

As children reach adolescence, they may be expected to become the caregivers of their ill parents or siblings even during acute phases of the illness. Their caregiving may inhibit their opportunities for social development and peer relationships. Children, like adults, may feel angry with their ill parent, or ill sibling, sometimes secretly wishing them dead. These secret feelings need to be expressed and resolved to alleviate the guilt that often accompanies them or the reactions to grief they experience if the loved one dies.

Chronic Illness in Adults

When serious chronic illness emerges in adulthood, it can occur in the primary family or in elderly parents. When it occurs in early adulthood it may interfere with people's ability to marry, have children, or become successful in their careers. In middle adulthood, illness can be perceived as disrupting the family and work systems. Mid-life is the time when major financial and other responsibilities for young children are completed. People are established in their roles and couples are often readying themselves for their retirement in good health. Plans that were put off for some time in the future seem close at hand, if not in place. Couples in mid-life are always aware of the potential for illness but their life scripts have its occurrence put off for older age.

With recent sophisticated medical technology, a first acute attack of an illness (cancer, heart attack) rarely ends in death. A couple will often have an opportunity to live for several, if not many, years with some quality of life. The quality of life is sometimes associated with their ability to change their definition of themselves to accommodate for the changes in their physical ability. Their quality of life is to some extent also dependent upon how their finances cover their medical and caregiving needs.

Caregiving can compromise their definitions of each other. Changing from an intimate couple relationship to a caregiving and care-receiving one is a difficult task for couples. If the spousal relationship is compromised by some loss of ability to do basic hygiene tasks, it may upset sexual and social boundaries. For example, in the case of sexuality, spouse caregivers of partners with dementia or Alzheimer's disease have reported finding particular distress with partners who make sexual overtures to them yet do not remember who they are or that they have participated at all (Litz, 1990). When the sexual intimacy of a relationship is changed by an illness, the couple or the caregiver may have to redefine their relationship from lovers to companions.

Caregiving may also change family's roles. For example, when there is a loss of control over body functions and the caregiving partner is responsible for diaper-changing and dressing responsibilities, the marital relationship may be perceived as being replaced by a parent-child dynamic. The ill person becomes ashamed of his or her inabilities, may withdraw or react angrily and/or may become despondent. Finding new meanings for accommodations to the relationship must be made in the context of communication between the partners. While dependency in physical needs may occur, the therapist can assist the partners to elicit maximum participation from the sick partner in family decisions and in any other ways that are possible. Encouraging participation of the ill spouse to the fullest extent throughout the course of the illness maximizes the quality of the relationship.

Gender factors have been known to play important parts in how care is given (Brok, 1992; Gwyther, 1990; Vinokur, 1990). Because of differing socialization, women tend to accept caregiving roles more readily than do men. Studies on post-cardiac incidents, indicate that women are better able to provide environments for their husbands to rest and recover because they have generally been responsible for the family chores (Badger, 1990). On the other hand, men tend to seek caregiving or housekeeping assistance from others when their wives are recuperating from acute illnesses. In less acute cases like Alzheimer's Disease, the caregiving responsibilities tend to be transferred over time (Gwyther, 1990). The caregivers most frequently sought are adult daughters although the healthcare system does provide some nursing and home health aide assistance, most often by women. Caregiving tends to isolate people and increases the caregiver's own risk for illness.

The status of a mid-life couple's social system in terms of other experiences with illness can affect their quality of life, if and when one member becomes chronically ill. If others in their peer group have had similar experiences, adjustment and support systems may be available. If adult children are close by, they may provide a replacement social support network. The least overall disruption in social activities or family gatherings, the easier the adaptation. Families can be encouraged to include the ill member in social situations wherever possible and discouraged from taking over all of the sick person's responsibilities.

In the case where these family and friend support networks are not available, medically-based peer groups (Heart clubs, Partners of People with Parkinson's Disease, etc.) offer a setting for families to reestablish themselves. These groups often provide a forum for the establishing of new friendships for both partners. By providing psycho-education about these support groups, a therapist or physician can assist the family to minimize their loneliness and isolation.

Chronic Illness in the Elderly

Chronic illness has often been defined as the illness of old age. It is also believed that if one lives long enough, one is expected to encounter a chronic illness, thus, leading individuals to assume that they will someday be ill. It is estimated that 85 percent of the elderly population in this country have a chronic illness, about half of those result in serious physical limitations (Schienle, 1894) and yet only about 5 percent of the population live in nursing homes (Stone, 1987). The life situation, experiences with loss, socio-economics and support systems of older people is often directly related to their stage of old age (65-75; 75-85; 85+) and their ability to cope with illness.

Belief systems about aging often affect the way families and the healthcare system respond to chronic illness in this later stage of life. If illness is defined as an anticipated, expected component of advancing age and elderly people are not expected to be able to care for themselves, then their care may be taken over by family members or the health system. If they themselves share this notion, they may relinquish themselves to the caregiving situation. Comments like "I'm old" are often synonymous with "I'm feeble" or "unable." These self-determinations may result in self-fulfilling prophecies that are often encouraged by well-meaning health care providers or children who become parents to their elderly parents. Furthermore, if it is acceptable for elderly persons to be unable to care for themselves and regain positions of health after a serious illness, then they may not be encouraged to do so. Yet, many older people do not succumb to these definitions and fight hard to maintain there independence and self-sufficiency. They recover and refuse care, sometimes to their families' distress.

The family's definition of itself as caregiver of its elderly members determines its willingness to give care, the style of caregiving and the ensuing effect. The caregiving needs of the elderly may be provided by a spouse, siblings or children. In long-term relationships, spouses usually have a vision about caring for one another in old age and are most comfortable when they can carry these out. Their scripts incorporate "till death do us part." Oftentimes, children interfere with these efforts in fear that the well parent's health is being irrevocably compromised. This interference may disrupt the lifetime promise and the well spouse caregiver responds to family pressure by giving up the role or keeping the family at a distance. Older spouses who give up responsibilities often feel that they have deserted their ill spouse and may become depressed and withdrawn. Other times, the well spouse caregiver continues the care, even though it may compromise their own health.

In some cases, spousal relationships were first entered into during this later life period and the role of caregiver and the expectations of families may already be imbalanced as their life scripts differ. Boundaries between the "new" well spouse and the birth of children or other relatives of the ill spouse often need to be established when serious illness occurs. Who makes the decisions, who does the caregiving, and where it will occur are problems that need to be resolved. Reconstituted families can become engaged in inevitable power struggles as they protect "their own." Environments that support older persons' belief systems and independent decision making wherever possible should be encouraged.

Often a couple has never expressed their feelings or their fears to one another about who will die first, or who will care for whom has never been expressed. These are difficult times for couples.

The Extended Family

In the case of children as caregivers, the extended family's proximity and responsibilities to their primary family may also influence how needs are met. Family of origin belief systems about what responsibilities adult children are "supposed" to have, how the different genders determine who does what, under what circumstances people should be institutionalized have implications to the delivery of care. The effects of caregiving an elderly parent may be profound on the family of the caregiver (spouse and children) especially when the ill parent comes to live with their child's family. Many marital relationships have deteriorated in the process of caregiving an elderly parent especially when the caregiving couple does not agree to the extent of responsibility or involvement.

General Caregiving Issues

Fairly recently, changes in hospital payment systems to systems of Diagnostic Related Groups (DRG) or managed care programs, has resulted in financial incentives for hospitals and medical personnel to release people in the shortest possible time. This has dramatically changed the face of caregiving. Professional home health care has emerged, along with the need for families to make provisions for its sick members more immediately. In these circumstances, people outside the family system invade the system constantly. Some actually enmesh with the system itself. Sociocultural factors such as extended family members living all over the country, reconstituted family systems, women in the workforce, and other such considerations have complicated the system further, making it more reliant on out-patient care. Yet, caregiving still remains a family issue.

Because of these changes in medical payment systems, changes in family proximity, and the aging of the population, recent research has been devoted to alternatives to the giving of care. Historically, care of infirmed people was the responsibility of the family, and where no family existed, the religious institutions. In families, men were responsible for the money to pay for the health needs of their ill and women for the hands-on care.

Caregiving has several meanings: love and intimacy, forgiveness, proving one's maturity, fulfilling obligations, and many others. Caregivers experience enormous frustration and sometimes "irrational anger, ambivalence, death wishes or escape fantasies" (Rolland, 1993). These intense feelings can result in distancing and guilt by the caregiver. Directing the caregivers intense, explosive frustrations at the illness rather than at the ill partner can diminish the guilt and bring the family closer together.

Summary and Conclusions

Historically, the primary care doctor in this country was a long-term friend of the family, lived in the neighborhood, and was an integral part of the social systems in which a family functioned. This trusted person had almost exclusive rights to the diagnosis and care of people who became ill in his practice (and it was usually a man). He engineered or directed care, which went far beyond medical treatment approaches, involved many family considerations and when the illness was long or serious the family often deemed him analogous to the "father." This model of treatment for people with illness rarely exists any longer. Medical personnel come in and out of family systems and play several different roles at different times. They rarely know much about the individual or the family system. In addition, acceptance of and understanding of ethnic and culturally-diverse ways of using or not using the health care system and the ways families care for their ill has also changed dramatically in this country. Yet, the support systems have not yet accommodated for these changes.

Chronic illness is not always easily diagnosed and treatments are complicated and often arduous, sometimes beyond the families' comprehensibility. Serious illnesses pose unmentionable threats of loss to family systems and their complexity results in imbalances in relationships that may change the player's roles, intimacy, boundaries, and life scripts.

A bio-psycho-social approach to helping families with chronic illness requires that therapists and medical practitioners create a new system of functioning with each other and the family. As Rolland (1993) so aptly put it, "therapists and couples need to understand the beliefs and multi-generational legacies that guide their constructions of meanings about health problems and their relationship to caregiving systems. Beliefs about normality, mind-body relationship and control, what caused an illness or what can affect its course, meanings or narratives developed around a health problem, and cultural/ethnic or gender-related beliefs are particularly significant" (p.15). They need also to begin to understand the medical progression and implications of the illness itself. Medical practitioners need to embrace families in their treatment of illness and expand their perspective from an individual medical model to a social systemic model. In this arena, families can begin to address the changes that must inevitably take place within the context of an illness. Changes that support the interpersonal relationships within the family, sustain intimacy and communication, create hope and foster coping in these families.

References

Atwood, J. (Ed.) (1996). *Family Scripts.* Chicago: Taylor & Francis.

Atwood, J. & Ruiz, J. (1993). Social constructionist therapy with the elderly. *Journal of Family Psychotherapy, 4*, 1, 1-31.

Badger, T. A. (1990). Men with cardiovascular disease and their spouses: Coping, health and marital adjustment. *Archives of Psychiatric Nursing,* IV (5), 319-324.

Bandura, A. (1977). Self-efficacy: Toward a unifying theory of behavioral change. *Psychological Review,* 84, 191-215.

Brok, A. J. (1992). Crises and transitions: Gender and life stage issues in individual, group, and couples treatment. *Psychoanalysis and Psychotherapy,* 10(1), 3-16.

Chekryn, J. (1984). Cancer recurrence: Personal meaning, communication and marital adjustment. *Cancer Nursing,* 7, 491-498.

Coyne, J. D., & DeLongis, A. (1986). Beyond social support: The role of social relationships in adaptation. *Journal of Consulting and Clinical Psychology,* 45, 456-460.

DiMatteo, M. R., & DiNicola, D. D. (1982). *Achieving Patient Compliance: The Psychology of the Medical Practitioner's Role.* New York: Pergamon.

Engel, G. L. (1977). The need for a new medical model: A challenge for biomedicine. *Science,* 196, 129-136.

Engel, G. L. (1980a). The clinical applications of the biopsychosocial model. *American Journal of Psychiatry,* 137, 535-544.

Epstein, L. H. (1984). The direct effect of compliance on health outcome. *Health Psychology,* 4(4), 385-393.

Gwyther, L. P. (1990). Letting go: Separation-Individuation in a wife of an Alzheimer's Patient. *The Gerontologist,* 30(5), 698-702.

Lachman, M. E. (1986). Personal control in later life: Stability, change and cognitive correlates. In P. B. B. MM Baltes (Eds.), *The Psychology of Control and Aging* Hillsdale, NJ: Erlbaum.

Litz, B. T.;. Z., A.M. & Davies, H.D. (1990). Sexual concerns of male spouses of female Alzheimer's disease patients. *Gerontologist,* 30, 113-116.

McDaniel, S. H., Hepworth, J & Doherty, W.J. (1992). *Medical Family Therapy: A Bio-Psychosocial Approach to Families with Health Problems.* New York: Basic Books, Inc.

Meyerowitz, B. E. (1983). Postmastectomy coping strategies and the quality of life. *Health Psychology,* 2, 117-132.

Mullan, F. (1983). *Vital Signs, a Young Doctor's Struggle with Cancer.* New York: Farrar, Straus, Giroux.

Phares, E. J. (1987). Locus of control. In R. J. Corsini (Eds.), *Concise Encyclopedia of Psychology.* New York: Wiley.

Rolland, J. S. (1993, December, 1993). Helping couples live with illness. *Family Therapy News,* p. 15, 26.

Sarafino, E. P. (1990). *Health Psychology: Biopsychosocial Interactions.* New York: John Wiley & Sons.

Schienle, D. R. &. E., J.M. (1894). Clinical intervention with older adults. In M. G.; S. Eisenberg L.C.; & Jansen, M.A. (Eds.), *Chronic Illness and Disability through the Life Span: Effects on Self and Family* (pp. 245-268). New York: Springer.

Shlain, L. (1979). Cancer is not a four-letter word. In C. A. Garfield (Eds.), *Stress and Survival: The Emotional Realities of Life-Threatening Illness.* St. Louis: C.V. Mosby.

Shontz, F. (1975). *The Psychological Aspects of Physical Illness and Disability.* New York: Macmillan Co.

Stone, R.; C., G. L; & Sangl, J. (1987). Caregiving of the frail elderly: A national profile. *Gerontologist*, 27, 616-629.

Swan, G.; Carmelli, D.; & Rosenman, R. (1986). Spouse-pair similarity on the California Psychological Inventory with reference to husband's coronary heart disease. *Psychosomatic Medicine*, 48(3/4), 185.

Turk, D. C., & Meichenbaum, D. (Ed.). (1991). *Adherence to Self-Care Regimens: The Patient's Perspective*. New York: Plenum.

Vinokur, A. D., & Kaplan, D.V. (1990). In sickness and in health: Patterns of social support and undermining in older married couples. *Journal of Aging and Health*, 2(2), 215-241.

3

Chronic Illness, Disability, Secondary Conditions, and the Culturally Diverse Family

Daniel W. Wong
Lucy Wong Hernandez

Abstract

This chapter provides readers with an understanding of how cultural factors play a significant role within families who have members with significant physical and mental health related issues such as chronic illnesses, disabilities, and secondary disabling conditions. The significance of how cultural factors contribute to the coping, adjusting, caring, and managing of family members who acquired chronic illnesses, disabilities, and secondary disabling conditions is of vital importance when assisting and providing therapy as a family therapy intervention. A summary of cultural competence skills recommendations for working with families from diverse cultural and ethnic backgrounds is also presented.

The challenge presented by a paradigm shift for future family therapy application in a culturally diverse society demands a better understanding and implementation of how family therapy and other disciplines in the human service and health care fields will adapt to the multiple issues presented by the people they serve.

This chapter will provide readers with an understanding of how cultural factors play a significant role within families who have members with significant physical and mental health-related issues such as chronic illnesses, disabilities, and secondary disabling conditions. The significance of how cultural factors will contribute to the coping, adjusting, caring, and managing of family members who acquired chronic illnesses, disabilities, and secondary disabling conditions is of vital importance when assisting and providing therapy as a family therapy intervention. A summary of cultural competence skills recommendations for working with families from diverse cultural and ethnic backgrounds will be presented.

Introduction

A demographic snapshot of the nation demonstrates that there has been a sizable growth in the proportion of multicultural populations living in the United States from 1980-2000. It is estimated that one in ten Americans was born outside the United States of America (U.S.A.) and an even larger proportion of culturally-diverse populations are projected for the year 2010. The constantly changing demographic and cultural configuration of the U.S.A. has alerted social service and health care professionals of the need to provide specific services to individuals from diverse cultural and ethnic backgrounds. These specific services should be offered in different ways according to the requirements imposed by cultural characteristics. The American Psychological Association (APA) and the American Counseling Association (ACA) have long been concerned with cultural issues and have developed specific guidelines for multicultural counseling (Casas, 1985). Recent legislation, in an effort to have a more equitable society, mandates practices relevant to the health and mental health cares, therapeutic and counseling practices, rehabilitation counseling, independent living services, and employment needs of persons with disabilities from diverse cultural and ethnic backgrounds to be culturally competent and culturally sensitive.

Understanding the sociocultural models of individuals with chronic illnesses, disabilities, and secondary conditions is of more than academic interest. Unless programs and services for individuals with chronic illnesses, disabilities, and secondary conditions are designed in a culturally appropriate way, the opportunity to make real and effective change is often lost. Cultural variables affecting these populations, such as values and beliefs, family structures, and attitudes towards illnesses and disabilities, are critically important to the outcome of the services provided. The intent is not to catalogue every known human variation and their perception of health-related challenges but rather to alert the practitioner to the fact that the ways in which chronic illnesses, disabilities, and secondary disabling conditions are conceptualized will have an impact on the manner in which professionals and therapeutic services are received, regarded, and able to serve their patients/clients effectively.

The Culturally-Diverse Family in America

The culturally-diverse family makes up the interconnected fabric of the American society. It is not a new socio-phenomenon rather it has been and still is the foundation of our richly diverse nation. As human service professionals, we have to recognize that individual and cultural diversity are important factors in any therapeutic intervention as they are in counseling, family therapy, psychotherapy, and rehabilitative services. These are equally important factors for health care professionals from different sectors. Since 1972 the APA has maintained that it is unethical for psychological service providers who are not competent in understanding persons of culturally-diverse backgrounds to provide such services to members of culturally-diverse minority groups (Korman, 1973). It has been indicated that, in the near future, the motives for working with and knowing about different cultural and ethnic groups will not be political liberalism or obligation. Rather, the motives will be enlightened self-interest and the wish and need to perform our work ethically and professionally.

The fact is that our society has become increasingly multicultural/ multi-ethnic and the self-interest of all will be served by developing skills and competencies needed when working with culturally-diverse populations. For human service professionals, the tasks are to better understand culturally diverse groups, to form conceptualizations of behavior that are applicable to diverse groups, and to promote the welfare of all human beings through education, teaching, and psychological therapeutic interventions. These tasks are neither simple nor new, but there is a special sense of the importance of addressing them because of rapid demographic population changes and the continuing differences on health and mental health inequities in well-being among diverse groups in the American society. The culturally-diverse family in America is not only diverse but also multi-dimensional, presenting an intellectual and ethical challenge to family therapists, counselors, and health care professionals.

Understanding the Definition of Culture

To understand the culturally-diverse family we need to understand culture in its broadest context. The concept of culture has been defined by social scientists in many different ways. According to Dillard (1983), "culture" consists of patterns of behaviors transmitted by symbols, values, and human products of a society that represents distinctive achievements of human groups. Culture can also be construed as the set of rules, shared belief systems, attitudes, and norms that promote stability and harmony within a social group (Gibbs & Huang, 1989; Kiselica, 1998). Culture regulates and organizes what a group feels, thinks, or does, but may be expressed individually in a variety of ways. Culture includes: familial roles; patterns of social and interpersonal communication; affective styles; values and ideals; spirituality and religion; habits of communication and artistic expressions; customs and norms; rituals and celebrations; and geographical and historical location. In sum, it is all that an individual and his/her family represents in their own worldview and culturally-based familial environment.

As in culture, it is important to also understand the meaning of ethnicity. Ethnic identity refers to people who share a common nationality, culture, language, and religious beliefs. An individual sense of self as a member of an ethnic group and the cultural attitudes and behaviors associated with that sense are very important to the uniqueness of the individual and the family. Therefore, we can say that culture is a set of distinctive behaviors, values, beliefs, and products that is expressive of a certain ethnic group and nationality (Cavina, 2005).

Despite the fact that cultural influences are in every fabric of society, they are often unrecognized or unappreciated, the importance of culture has been noted by many scholars especially those involved in cross-cultural research. Albert (1988) has examined several factors that can lead to the neglect of cultural variables. They include lack of contact and experience with other cultures, the need to simplify rather than complicate perceptions within a cultural context, fears that lead to stereotyping others because of cultural backgrounds, ethnocentric bias, and equating diversity with elitism. These factors are often at the root of much emotional conflict within and between individuals including among different professional fields and should be avoided.

Family Structure and Its Culture

In today's continuously changing world, societal norms and demands concerning the family's roles and functions are in a process of rapid transformation. Nevertheless, the family unit still constitutes the main framework in which the individual grows and develops. Since the family is an integral component of society, it can be expected to show much variation across cultures. Although anthropologists have drawn attention to the cross-cultural diversity of family types and relationships, it seems that psychologists tend to undervalue the importance of variety in family patterns while they remain concerned with other issues related to the client/patient. Nonetheless, one may observe a growing interest in the understanding of the impact of culture and ethnicity upon family dynamics, particularly during challenging developmental stages such as adolescence and in the later stage of life as in old-aging.

It is well-documented that there are many differences in family dynamics between cultural and ethnic groups in the United States. These differences manifest themselves in different ways in the organization of the family, however, they are all based on the culture and levels of acculturalization of family members. In spite of this important factor, socially and emotionally-matured family members, and in particular those who are of a younger age are expected to stay loyal to the family culture and under the guidance of their parents or elderly family members.

Culture continues to be a strong force in family dynamics and how they perceive themselves among their cultural groups and outside their cultural groups. Behavior and self-perception are influenced by how the family organizes around their culture. Culture remains true but the challenges of "what to do" to become socially included and accepted by the majority dissipated with time. Families of diverse cultures demand respect and fair treatment from all sectors of society and most importantly from family health care systems including family therapists, counselors, and other professionals concerned with biopsychosocial family issues.

Learning about Family Culture from the Clients' Stories

It is important for professionals to learn about family culture; however this can be a difficult task if professionals do not pay particular attention to the "cultural clues" that are given through family stories narrated by the client and/or patient and their family members. Attention should be given to body language, culturally-based gestures, and linguistic ability because through them "stories" are told. As we know, some cultures are more expressive than others and some demonstrate a deep respect towards professionals more than others, which bring an interesting variable on how the client story will be told. The professional worker can be culturally-viewed as someone with authority and able to resolve all the problems and cure the person from any illness. This perception should be clarified with open communication and positive patient-professional relationship. A family member's story can provide all the signs to encourage the professional to conduct further exploration for possible intervention by using culturally-based skills that can encourage the client/patient to reveal more than what is being said and shown during the therapeutic interaction. The family culture and its dynamic can present a challenge if it is not approached in a culturally competent manner. Whenever appropriate, genograms and other theories such as narrative theories techniques can prove to be beneficial to learn more from the family's culture and help them in a more effective way. Additionally, the biopsychosocial systems approach to working with clients experiencing health issues is also beneficial. In this form of therapy, the focus is on the role medical illness and disability play in the client's emotional life and in the client's relationships with family members and with health care professionals. It is of vital importance for service providers to understand the medical and psychosocial aspects of the medical illness, in some cases chronic and the disability, in most cases permanent and progressive.

Defining Chronic Illness, Disability and Secondary Conditions

Chronic Illness. Individuals living with a long-lasting health condition (also called a chronic illness) encounter many challenges. These challenges include health-related issues (including secondary conditions due to the primary condition) that confront the individual; family members and caregivers coping with these challenges; negative attitudes that prevent full participation in community services and integration into society; and negative impact on the family's financial status due to loss of wages and possible employability.

It is important to review the long standing definitions of illness. There are two types of illnesses: acute and chronic. Acute illnesses depending on its severity (like a cold or the flu) are usually over relatively quickly. Chronic illnesses, though, are long-lasting health conditions (the word "chronic" comes from the Greek word *chronos*, meaning time) that may even have consequences of secondary conditions that are related to the primary chronic condition (such as diabetes and limb amputation).

Having a chronic condition does not necessarily mean that an illness is critical or dangerous—although some chronic illnesses, such as cancer and AIDS, can be life-threatening. Chronic illnesses can also include conditions like asthma, arthritis, cardiovascular diseases, and diabetes. Although the symptoms of a chronic illness might "go away" or go on remission with proper medical care, usually a person will continue to have the underlying condition—even though their medical treatments contribute to the possibility of feeling completely healthy and well much of the time.

Disability. The Americans with Disabilities Act (ADA) defines the term disability as it relates to "an individual with a disability is a person who has: (A) a physical or mental impairment that substantially limits one or more of the major life activities of such individual; (B) has a record of such an impairment; or (C) is being regarded as having such an impairment" (ADA, 2008).

Secondary Conditions. Secondary conditions, an expression of the medical term "comorbidity" are medical, physical, cognitive, emotional, and psychological consequences to which persons with chronic illnesses and disabilities are more susceptible. In other words, a secondary condition is *"any condition to which a person is more susceptible by virtue of having a primary disabling condition"* (Nosek, 2004). However, a *secondary condition* adds three dimensions not fully captured by the previous term *comorbidity*. It includes: 1) non-medical events such as social isolation; 2) conditions that affect the general population such as obesity and diabetes, but which more greatly affect people with disabling conditions; 3) problems that arise during the lifespan, like inaccessible preventive medical screening among many other medical procedures; and 4) lack of access and affordability to therapeutic services (Nosek, 2004; Patrick, 1997). The serious impact of these issues of secondary conditions on diverse populations has prompted the Centers for Disease Control and Prevention (CDC) to set a national agenda as one of the goals of *Healthy People 2010* to eliminate well-documented health disparities and differences that occur among segments of the population, including gender, sexual orientation, race, culture and ethnic background, education, socioeconomic status, environmental risks, and geographic location (Healthy People 2010, 2001). In addition, all of these variables play an important role on how secondary conditions are prevented, diagnosed, and managed. The impact of secondary conditions on the person and the family can be devastating requiring biopsychosocial knowledge of the condition for effective intervention by the family therapist, counselor, or health care professional.

Cultural Perspectives of Chronic Illness, Disability, and Secondary Conditions

It is important to note that different cultures may have a different perception, understanding, expectation, and mode of treatment for chronic illnesses and disabilities including secondary conditions. They may also have cultural-based opinions and expectations of professionals in the medical field mental health and human services.

One aspect that is constant for all cultures and ethnic groups is that: good health is an interest of people of all cultures. However, the ways in which various cultures view, react to, cope, adjust, and treat chronic illness, disability, and secondary conditions has distinctive variations. It may be said that acceptance and perception of these conditions are culturally determined. By identifying how various cultures react, cope, and perceive chronic illness, disability, and secondary conditions the human service providers such as counselors and family therapists can also identify specific skills and help-seeking behavior of individuals from diverse cultural and ethnic backgrounds. Recent studies point out that the degree of acceptance of chronic illness, disability, and secondary condition may influence an individual and his or her family members on how they function as a family unit in order to effectively cope with this situation (Wong-Hernandez & Wong, 2001).

A challenge for family therapy and counseling is that it is almost impossible to understand the meaning of behavior unless one knows of the cultural values of the client/patient or family receiving the therapy services. Even the definition of "family" differs greatly from group to group. The dominant American (Anglo) definition focuses on the intact nuclear family, whereas in other cultures there is no such thing as "nuclear family." To some cultural groups family means strong, tightly knit that could be three or four-generational family, which also includes godparents and old friends or extended family as in the case of some cultures such as Italians, Spaniards, and Hispanic/Latino, among others. African-American families focus on an even wider network of kin and community all equally important to their meaning of family. Asian families include all ancestors tracing back to the beginning of time, and all descendants, or at least male ancestors and descendents, reflecting a sense of time heavily rooted on ethnic affiliation that is almost inconceivable to most other Americans (McGoldrick, Giordano & Garcia-Petro, 2005). These are important cultural characteristics that need to be clearly understood when we ask or try to identify: Who is the family?; What are the family members' roles?; Who makes the decisions?; and Who takes responsibilities?

The following factors have been identified by other scholars to be associated with the perception and coping mechanism of chronic illnesses, disabilities, and secondary conditions among people from diverse cultural and ethnic backgrounds. As an example of two cultural groups that are rapidly increasing among the fabrics of the American society who are classified as Hispanics or Latinos and Asians we find very culturally-specific characteristics that demand our attention as human service and health care providers.

The Culturally Based Well-Defined Gender Roles

It is well-documented in the social sciences that most men, especially Hispanics and Asians have been culturally taught that it is their responsibility to provide for their families and being strong is considered an important male attribute. Acceptance of a chronic illness, disability, and secondary condition may therefore be more difficult for them than for clients/patients who perceive their roles less stringently based on gender (Wong-Hernandez & Wong, 2001). Women also have their cultural designated roles within the family. In most cultures the woman is the caregiver, the protective force, and the administrator of family affairs as well as the anchor for stability and support among family members. In today's society the role of women has changed significantly and these changes also impacts women from diverse cultures as it does on issues of working outside the home to contribute to the financial household while still holding all their other ascribed roles and responsibilities as daughter, wife, mother, sister, and friend.

Migration has also defined the gender role among cultural groups. Migration is so disruptive to the individual and the family that it seems to add an entire extra stage to the life cycle for those who must negotiate it (Hernandez & McGoldrick, 2005). Adjusting to a new cultural environment is not a single event, but rather a prolonged development process that affects family members differently, depending on their life cycle phase when they are going through the process of assimilation and acculturalization.

Attitude toward Life Events

The perception of chronic illness, disability, and secondary conditions among Hispanics and Asians may be affected by what many researchers identify as a culturally-based attitude of resignation and acceptance of life problems. There may be less inclination to question, complain, or strive for change than among people from other cultural backgrounds. This rather passive attitude for both cultures should not be misunderstood with lack of interest or feelings of guilt and resignation. It should be understood from a more cultural-religious-spiritual perspective of accepting the things that cannot be avoided or changed. It is more likely to find that families in these two cultural groups are not resisting or fighting back the destiny of the individual and the family. Appreciation of cultural variability leads to a radically new conceptual model of clinical intervention. Helping a person or family achieve a stronger sense of self may require resolving internalized negative cultural attitudes or cultural conflicts within the family, between the family and the community, or in the wider context in which the family is embedded. A part of the clinical process involves identifying and consciously selecting cultural and ethnic values we wish to reinforce.

A Cohesive, Protective, Family-Oriented Society

Researchers agree that culturally-diverse family members play important roles in the therapeutic and rehabilitation process and outcomes of the services being delivered. At times, these cultural characteristics have been viewed by many practitioners as overprotective and paternalistic, and limiting the client's full and active participation. With a better understanding of the cultural-based approach the therapist or service provider will utilize these variables to the best advantage for the client/patient and his/her family. Important decisions of issues related to disclosures, acceptance of treatment modality, and follow-ups in most cases need to involve the responsible family members, at times including the extended family and familial links as well.

Impact of Religious Views

Religion plays an important role in the definition, response, and acceptance of chronic illness and disability for a large population among culturally-diverse clients. As an example, in the Hispanic worldview, illness and disability is often seen as a punishment for one's sins or for the sins that one's parents may have committed in life. Among the Asian cultures these challenges may be perceived as part of the family's "karma" or destiny before entering another level of existence based on their religious beliefs. It is important for counselors, therapists, and other mental health practitioners to understand that such a "theological etiology" may be ascribed to the acceptance and understanding of chronic illnesses and disabilities by many Hispanic and Asian clients/patients and their families. This could also explain what is perceived by professionals as apathy toward the therapeutic intervention from these two specific groups.

Perceptions of Physical and Mental Disabilities

Physical and mental disabilities have a high prevalence among culturally-diverse individuals. For Hispanic populations physical disabilities among working age groups (16-60 years old) occurs very frequently in most cases due to their involvement in high risk occupational accidents and hazardous contamination as in the case of persons working for the farming industries. Mental chronic illnesses are associated with the inability to assimilate a new culture with the consequence of bouts of anxiety and depression complicated by lifestyles and the effects of alcohol and drug dependency for some individuals.

Canino, Earley and Rogler (1980) have indicated in their research of the mental health status of Hispanics that this population experiences a greater array of potentially stress-inducing events than do other populations and thus have higher risk for mental health problems. Several aspects of the transition from one society to another apparently constitute hazardous situations leading to increased risk of psychiatric episodes of long-term hospitalizations. In these cases a deep psychosocial analysis of the individual and the family must have cultural context for appropriate culturally-based intervention.

The Impact of Chronic Illnesses, Disabilities, and Secondary Conditions on the Family

The impact of chronic illnesses disabilities and secondary conditions on families has been researched extensively. However, the impact of secondary disabling conditions has not been fully studied and understood. It is important to recognize that an estimated 54 million persons in the United States or nearly 20 percent of the population currently live with some type of a medical diagnosed disability. The direct medical and indirect annual costs associated with disability are more than $300 billion, which is over 4 percent of the gross domestic product (U.S. Department of Health and Human Services, 2005).

As indicated by *Healthy People 2010*, this cost includes over $160 billion in medical care expenditures and over $155 billion in lost productivity costs (Healthy People 2010, 2001). These numbers indicate a significant public health and economic burden to society as well as the need for suitable and sensitive health care interventions and preventive methods that can lessen this economic impact and afford healthy quality of life to persons with chronic illnesses and disabilities and their family members.

Traditionally, health promotion as a preventive method for secondary conditions for persons with chronic illnesses and disabilities has not been a significant area of interest on the part of the general health care and mental health service fields. Today, researchers, funding agencies, health care providers, rehabilitation professionals and persons with disabling conditions are leading the efforts to prioritize future research studies and establish higher-quality and equitable health care, rehabilitation, prevention of secondary conditions, and bio-psychosocial interventions for all persons facing these challenges. It is important to note the paradigm shift from chronic illness, disability prevention, and rehabilitation to prevention of secondary conditions and promotion of health and wellness including mental health. There has also been a shift towards the need for further cultural, ethnic, and environmentally relevant interventions as well as research studies on these topics, which address the centrality of health to quality of life of millions of Americans with chronic illnesses and disabilities (Rimmer, 1999). Most importantly, the involvement of the families with respect to these interventions will play a significant role for prevention of secondary conditions and the improvement of the quality of life of the individual and the family.

Chronic illnesses, disabilities, and secondary conditions will affect the entire family with respect to health and mental health care of the individual with the condition, possible negative economical impact on the family, and psychological stress that all family members have to endure. The coping and adjustment process to these issues may have enormous consequences for all members of the family. The onset of a chronic illness, a disability, or a secondary condition within a family may affect the family differently depending on who has acquired the chronic illness or disability and what the family role was for this person. The perception of the condition may also influence how the family will intervene and care for the family member. The issues of psychiatric illness are perceived by many culturally-diverse families as one of the most difficult to manage and one with the most negative stigma among that particular cultural/ethnic group and society at large.

As indicated earlier in the section covering well-defined gender roles, a characteristic of most cultures worldwide is that a man always considers himself the dominant partner or the bread-winner of the family. They have been culturally taught about their male-role responsibilities and being strong is considered an important male attribute. Acceptance of chronic illnesses, disabilities, and secondary conditions may, therefore be more difficult for the men of these patriarch-oriented cultures than for men from other cultures with less strictly gender-based roles. These individuals may have difficulties in allowing their spouses to assist them on making decisions day after day with respect to health care, financial issues, and other important family matters. This family role conflict may jeopardize the harmony of the family and impose a substantial psychological stress on the family as family roles and responsibilities may shift.

These stressors may have a negative result and many dire consequences to the family, such as psychosomatic syndromes, depression, headache, backache, alcohol and substance abuse, lost of employment, traffic accidents, and family separation among many others. Women have their cultural-based roles well-defined but for most it is expected that they will endure in "silence" in any challenges of health and mental health conditions. This expectation may be due to the fact that in many cultures women may not be expected to be financial contributors or leaders to their family but rather occupy their passive role based on gender (i.e., daughter, wife, mother, etc.). While these outdated expectations are rejected in Western society, we need to be cognizant that they are very valid among other cultural and ethnic societies.

According to Ware and Kleinman (1992), chronic illnesses, disabilities, and secondary conditions are not simply the "natural" unfolding of an exclusively biological process; its course is also social. They argued that there are meanings in reference to the concept of the social course of chronic illnesses. One important belief and notion is that the severity of symptomatology is influenced by aspects of the social environment. Persons with chronic illnesses, disabilities, and secondary conditions from diverse cultural and ethnic backgrounds may encounter and could be subjected to more negative events because of discrimination and marginalization from the society at large, which will further intensify and impair their adjustment and coping with their conditions.

Ware and Kleiman (1992) also stated that this "sociosomatic" formulation, as a dialectic relationship between the individual and the society plays a critical role on improving or further impairing the individual's recovery and coping with his or her chronic illness and/or disability. The psychosocial aspect of the health-related condition is affected by multiple variables such as society perception, racial, cultural and ethnic biases, the build environment, the quality and expectation of services, and the patient/client relationship with the service provider.

Recommendations for Training Supervisors, Supervisees, Counselors, Therapists, and Other Health Care Professionals

The need for multicultural sensitivity, cultural competence, and understanding of the implications of chronic illnesses, disabilities, and secondary conditions is critical for the success of family therapists, counseling, and other related therapeutic services in the health care disciplines. It is essential to examine multicultural training as a cultural competence tool that will enhance the client-counselor/therapist work relationship and service outcomes. Cultural competence is understood as having the capacity and skills to function effectively as an individual, organization, or service provider within the context of the cultural beliefs and practices and understand the needs presented by the client/patient, family, and their community. It is a conscious and social reaction to do what is culturally appropriate and putting all biases, if any, aside. Cultural sensitivity is a cognitive reaction that involves knowing that cultural differences as well as similarities exist, without assigning values (i.e., better or worse, right or wrong) to those cultural differences.

Culturally-appropriate supervision from a supervisee's and client's perspective is critical in the delivery of therapeutic interventions. Supervisors at the academic levels or at internship agency sites should be encouraged to identify issues related to individuals from diverse cultures and ethnic backgrounds from two different perspectives: the students in training and the clients receiving services. This practice will allow both supervisors and supervisees to understand cultural implications and dispel any misconceptions or possible barriers that interfere with possible treatments. This will also allow the supervisors and the supervisees to honor each other's cultural upbringing and worldview.

Miles (1999) in defining the counselor and/or therapist's role has indicated that it is hardly the therapist's job to try to change a client's fundamental cultural beliefs. To attempt this might be seen as unprofessional conduct and unethical. Ethical principles in relationship with clients demonstrate respect for the cultural and religious values of those they serve and refrain from imposing their own values and beliefs on those served. It is recommended to avoid imposition of theology and cultural values on those served or supervised. Yet for most therapists and counselors their work is more than a bag of techniques and gadgets to be used at anytime. The therapist and counselor cannot avoid some engagement with client's efforts to make sense of their chronic illnesses, disabilities, and secondary condition, or those of their family members. To listen attentively and with cultural-based understanding requires the competent therapist to have some broad awareness of the range of human beliefs about the chronic illness and disability biopsychological areas, and at least an outward tolerance of someone that may seem personally different and unpleasant. One benefit of studying cultural aspects further is that it may be possible to hint at paths that would take clients toward a more positive position within their own belief systems.

Hird, Cavalieri, Dulko, Felice, & Ho (2001) provided recommendations for multicultural supervisors to improve cross-cultural supervision that include: a) increased self awareness; b) continued professional development; c) continued practical experience; d) joining multicultural professional organizations; e) peer supervision; f) joint attendance to multicultural workshops by supervisors and supervisees, and; g) use of evaluation tools that assess the multicultural competence of service providers, supervisors and supervisees alike. In clinical interventions, standards of multicultural competencies involve identifying major life events, relationships, and cultural contexts that influence professional identity as expressed in human service provision. Multicultural competencies take into consideration multiple elements of cultural and ethnic differences, social conditions, systems, and justice issues without imposing their own perspectives. A culturally-sensitive family therapist or counselor will demonstrate competent use of self-expertise and professional function, which include: emotional availability, cultural humility, appropriate self-disclosure, positive use of power and authority, a non-anxious and judgmental presence, and clear and responsible boundaries (Wong-Hernandez & Wong, 2002 and Stone, 2005).

Training Culturally-Competent Therapists

As indicated in the recommendations above, to serve culturally-diverse American families effectively, marriage and family therapists, and other counseling professionals need to develop the highest possible level of cultural competence. Although definitions differ somewhat across mental health disciplines, cultural competence is typically conceptualized as involving the three main areas as proposed by Sue et al (1992). First, therapists awareness—of own culture and its specific impact on the formation of values and biases; second therapists knowledge—of the worldview of the culturally-different client and his/her family; third, therapists behaviors—the use of culturally appropriate treatment strategies and interventions. All three areas are important to a therapist's educational and professional development and a variety of ideas have been proposed in this chapter to help supervisors and educators train culturally-competent student family therapists and counselors.

In the areas of therapist and counselor awareness, Hardy and Laszloffy (1992) advised supervisors to help trainees appreciate the role of culture in their lives through cultural genograms and "storytelling" of their own ethnic history. Similarly, Coleman (1997) suggested using qualitative-based portfolios to allow students to discuss and document their experiences as they become more culturally aware of self and others. In terms of therapist knowledge, clinicians have usually been instructed using historical accounts of the group's experience in the United States and/or popular representations of the ethnic culture (e.g., movies, books, music, etc.). This information helps therapists begin to understand how culture, ethnicity, religion, education, racism, and other contextual factors affect the family, and how these factors combine ecosystemically to result in a particular worldview (Falicov, 1995). Portfolios have been advocated a means of evaluating therapist development in this area as well (Coleman, 1997); yet the more common measure of a therapist's understanding of a culturally-different client seems to be his/her ability to behave in a manner that is responsive and respectful to the client's cultural worldview (Ridley et al, 1994). Unfortunately, this leads beginning therapists and their supervisors to the imprecision and subjectivity associated with the third area of therapist development—therapist behavior. Ridley et al (1994) observed that the inherent difficulty in training culturally-competent therapists and counselors is due, in part, to the lack of clear behavioral indicators of therapist competence or sensitivity. Because of the shortage of clinical research in this area it has been difficult to make reliable judgments about the treatment strategies and therapist behaviors that are representative of culturally-competent therapy with families from diverse cultural and ethnic backgrounds. Consequently, supervisors are often left without clear standards for training and evaluating trainees, which can leave trainers and therapists feeling frustrated and confused.

The purpose is that in an effort to facilitate the training and evaluation of culturally-competent therapists, a content analysis should be conducted to better understand the available literature regarding family therapy treatment with culturally-different families. While considering the within-group diversity found among culturally-diverse families the purpose of any type of cultural competence training should be to avoid the "myth of sameness" or ethnic group homogeneity (Wong & Wong-Hernandez, 2007). Given the diversity in demographic factors, such as family structure, socioeconomic status, and national origin, an entire set of therapeutic guidelines cannot be expected to apply to every family of a culturally-diverse origin. Nevertheless, for training purposes, it is important to establish a "starting point" standard for defining and evaluating culturally-competent therapy with the culturally-diverse American family that will take into consideration the family individuality.

In training culturally-competent therapists, marriage and family therapists or counselors and in particular medical family therapists need to go beyond the typical practices of looking at culturally diversity as something that is very different and not related to the majority of society.

Marriage and family educators and supervisors need to assume positions of leadership by transforming their programs and trainees to reflect a deep, active, systemic commitment to both diversity and social justice. It is through this type of transformation and training techniques that programs become truly ready to prepare all student therapists to advocate for equity in a diverse and often unfair society.

Training Culturally-Competent Health Care Providers

Patient-centered and cultural competence training models have been promoted extensively in recent years as approaches to improving health care quality and train health care providers. There has been a historical evolution of both concepts demonstrating that early conceptual models focused on how health care providers and patients interact at the interpersonal level, while later models were expanded to consider how patients were treated by the health care system as a whole. These training models are compared at both the interpersonal and health care system levels to demonstrate similarities and differences. Although the two concepts have grown out of separate traditions, each with its own focus, many of the core features of patient-centeredness and cultural competence are the same. Each training model holds promise for improving the quality of health care for individual patients' communities and diverse populations. Although the two approaches to train health care providers and improve health care delivery have grown out of the separate traditions they have significant similarities and implications for improving health care quality at the level of interpersonal care and at the health-system level.

Patient-centeredness originated in the late 1960s as a way of characterizing how physicians and other health care providers should interact and communicate with patients on a more personal level. However, during the academic experience of this, professional training of cultural competence was by far not mentioned as an important contributor to the patient-health care-professional relationship. Some of the core features of this training model include: understanding the patient as a unique person, exploring the patient's experience of illness, finding common ground regarding treatment through shared decision making, and an emphasis on building the doctor-patient and nurse-patient relationship. In essence, patient-centeredness involves perceiving and evaluating health care from the patient's perspective and adapting care to meet the needs and expectations of patients. This technique would be totally impossible if one does not have the cultural competence and sensitivity to truly understand the patient and his/her family's culturally-based worldview.

The important issue of cultural competence in health care emerged years later than patient-centeredness. The term "cultural competence" did not begin to appear consistently in the medical literature until the early 1990s. The primary impetus for this movement in the last decade has been the demonstration of pervasive racial and ethnic disparities in health care, most notable publicized in the 2002 IOM report, *Unequal Treatment*. The report and its underlying research gave rise to an explosion of interest in culturally-competent health care and appropriate training to achieve this knowledge.

Cultural competence training for health care professionals must also be considered in the context of decade-old initiatives to eliminate the cultural and linguistic barriers between health care providers and patients, which can interfere with the effective delivery of health care services. Sometimes described as "cross-cultural," "transcultural," "multicultural," or "culturally sensitive," these efforts were initially targeted at immigrant or refugee populations with limited English proficiency and exposure to Western cultural norms. Some efforts to train professionals to work effectively with this specific culturally-diverse population had the potential to emphasize culture-centered rather than patient-centered care, which proved to be a drawback. That is, these training efforts emphasized patients as members of ethnic or cultural groups, rather than as individuals with unique experiences and perspectives, possibly leading providers to stereotype and make inappropriate assumptions and ignoring the unique differences among subcultural groups by lumping all members of a subcultural group under the same regional cultural block (i.e. Hispanics from different Latin American countries).

Due to research and development in the health care field, the cultural competence movement tempered this emphasis on specific cultural groups and expanded in scope to include all people from diverse cultural and ethnic groups, particularly those most affected by racial disparities in the quality of health care.

Innovative cultural competence training for health care professionals need to borrow from different disciplines in order to become "social-justice" appropriate and eliminate the barriers that diversity may present as a challenge to the profession. One of the most important elements of cultural competence training is reinforcing the individuality and respect for the patient's worldview, cultural values, and beliefs as well as that of the entire family. Understanding the importance of family members' input and their involvement in decision making is also equally important when implementing culturally-competent techniques in the health care provision.

Training Recommendations for Professional Programs for a Better Understanding of the Culturally Diverse Family

A culturally-appropriate professional training program should begin by taking the necessary steps towards defining one's ethnic and cultural identity, investigating the trainees own racial, ethnic, and cultural heritage by: paying attention to their cultural roots; the social location of their upbringing; ethnic ties and cultural context; and the movement in and out of successive social locations and cultural contexts in the trainee's life journey. The following are culturally-based recommendations for training:

1. The attitudes and self-awareness of the trainees should be evaluated to determine what training programs should be developed to provide cultural sensitivity training to them in reference to maximizing their respect toward diverse cultures and issues related to chronic illnesses, disabilities, and secondary conditions.

2. Students and trainees should be required to demonstrate self-reflective awareness and provide culturally-appropriate therapeutic assessment and interventions to patients/clients and their family members and or significant others. The assessment should include the immediate crisis, which challenges the patient/client's well-being; the relationship to illness and disability and the body image; the patient/client's connection to personal, cultural, spiritual resources, and the theological and spiritual issues expressed by the individual during the therapeutic dialogue.

3. Training models with respect to the understanding of the implications of chronic illnesses, disabilities, and secondary conditions among diverse cultures should be requirements in any curriculum for educational training. This requirement will enable trainees to develop skills to understand various cultural-based practices that are relevant to the patient/client and his/her family's psychological aspects in regard to coping and make necessary adjustment with the challenges at hand.

4. Trainees should be trained to understand the difference and similarities among various cultures with respect to their understanding and practice of social and medical models. This will allow a better understanding and enhance the patient/client-therapist work relationship and contribute to positive therapeutic outcomes.

5. It is critically important to identify the patient/client's and their immediate family members' strengths and struggles and their spiritual and cultural context. Equally important is to validate the various aspects of the crisis, including the role of culture that could sustain the person or could aggravate the struggle.

6. To develop an appropriate intervention plan based on the ability to communicate cross-culturally, to choose a specific therapeutic focus and to maintain an attitude that is culturally sensitive and valued.

7. Working and empowering families who have family members with chronic illnesses, disabilities, and secondary conditions is a critical step to encourage families to identify their needs and strength in order for them to assist their family members more as caregivers effectively. Family members need to have an understanding of medical information and the implications of the chronic illnesses, disabilities, and secondary conditions and how it may affect other family members. Family members will need to learn how to access and utilize community resources available to maximize the coping and adjustment for their family members with chronic illnesses and disabilities (Atwood & Weinstein, 2001).

8. Training modules should enable students, trainees, and professionals to demonstrate the ability to communicate effectively across a diversity of cultures, ethnicities, and spiritual traditions; understand and respect cultural identities with their norms and behaviors, values and beliefs, different worldviews and different spiritual frames of reference; provide appropriate and specific-to-the-case guidance, support, and presence with an awareness of cultural and contextual issues.

9. Awareness of cultural contexts will enhance cultural differences focus on a variety of aspects such as: relation of individual with family and community before and after onset of chronic illness and/or disability; different use of time (monochromic or polychromic); different use of space (proximity tolerance); focus on content or context priority (value placed on content or on relational context); communication styles (direct or indirect); age, gender, familial role, and socially-accepted ability to make independent choices; boundaries between personal and public; public image and self-image ("face" and self).

10. The motivation of becoming culturally competent benefits the trainees beyond the need for a successful career. It must be clear for every student, trainee, and professional that it is absolutely, positively impossible for anyone to understand clearly, empathize accurately, and care skillfully for patients/clients and families, if one is "culturally clueless." This would lead to ethnocentrism, or the conscious or unconscious assumption that an individual's worldviews are the rule for the rest of the world. The opposite of being "culturally clueless" is to become "culturally competent."

The journey of understanding the culturally-diverse client/patient and the family is a lifelong journey, and the destination is the process itself. The journey to cultural competence in order to have a better understanding of the implications of chronic illnesses' and disabling conditions' impact on the family is a challenging one for the service provider and for the individual and family presenting the challenges. There are four stages to mark this journey: cultural encapsulation; cultural awareness; cultural sensitivity; and cultural competence. The prerequisite is cultural humility while thinking critically, and the ability to remain open, imaginative, receptive, and curious. Becoming culturally competent will enable the trainees to identify the six obstacles to the delivery of effective cultural appropriate services: confusion, defensiveness, fear, ignorance, pain, and the attachment to one's particular view.

The future professionals of a culturally-diverse American society will need to be willing to embrace the new, respect the richness of cultural diversity, engage in an intercultural exchange that is ethical, spiritual, emotional, and deeply challenging.

References

Albert, R. D. (1988). The place of culture in modern psychology. In P. Bronstein & K. Quina (Eds.), *Teaching a Psychology of People.* 12-20. Washington, D.C.: American Psychological Association.

Americans with Disabilities Act (2008). Retrieved March 1, 2008 from U.S. Department of Justice (*www.usdoj.gov/crt/ada/pubs/ada.txt*).

Atwood, J. & Weinstein, E. (2001). *Family Practice, Medical Family Therapy: A Collaboration of Dialogue.* New York: J. Wiley & Sons.

Canino, I.A., Early, B.I., & Rogler, L.H. (1980). *Hispanics in New York City: Stress and Mental Health.* New York, NY: Fordham University Hispanics Research Center.

Casas, J. M. (1985). The status of racial and ethnic minority counseling: A training perspective. In P. Pedersen (Ed), *Handbook of Cross-Cultural Counseling and Therapy* 267-274. Wesport, CT: Greenwood.

Cavina, A. P. (2005). Multicultural Competencies in the Practice of Supervision. Multicultural Competencies Task Force.

Coleman, H. L. K. (1997). Portfolio assessment of multicultural counseling competence. In D. B. Pope-Davis & H. L. K. Coleman (Eds.). *Multicultural Counseling Competencies: Assessment, Education and Training, and Supervision.* Thousand Oaks, CA: Sage.

Dillard, J.M. (1983). *Multicultural Counseling.* Chicago, IL: Nelson-Hall.

Falicov, C. J. (1995). Training to think culturally: A multidimensional comparative framework. *Family Process,* 34, 373-388.

Friedlander, M. L., & Kaul, T. J. (1983). Preparing clients for counseling: Effects of role induction on counseling process and outcome. *Journal of College Student Personnel,* 24, 207-214.

Gibbs, J. T., & Huang, L. N. (1989). A conceptual framework for assessing and treating minority youth. In J. T. Gibbs & L. N. Huang (Eds.), *Children of Color: Psychological Interventions with Minority Youths.* San Francisco, CA: Jossey-Bass.

Grier, W. H. & Cobbs, P. M. (1968). *Black Rage.* New York: Basic.

Hardy, K. V. & Laszloffy, T. A. (1992). Training racially sensitive family therapists: Context, content, and contact. *Families in Society,* 73, 364-370.

Healthy People 2010. (2001). *Disability and Secondary Conditions.* Centers for Disease Control and Prevention. National Institute on Disability and Rehabilitation and Research, US Department of Education. V.1.

Hernandez, M. & McGoldrick, M. (2005). Migration and family life cycle. In B. Carter & M. McGoldrick (Eds), *The Expanded Family Life Cycle.* Boston, MA: Allyn & Bacon.

Hird, J. S., Cavalieri, C.E., Dulko, J.P., Felice, A.A.D., & Ho, T.A. (2001). Vision and realities: Supervisee perspectives of multicultural supervision. *Journal of Multicultural Counseling & Development*, 29(2), 114-130.

Korman, M. (Ed.). (1973). *Level and Patterns of Professional Training in Psychology.* Washington, DC: American Psychological Association.

McGoldrick, M.; Giordano, J.; & Garcia-Petro, N. (2005). *Ethnicity and Family Therapy* (Ed.) 3rd Ed. New York, NY: The Guilford Press.

Miles, M. (1999). Some influences of religions on attitudes towards disabilities and people with disabilities. In R. Levitt (Ed.) Cross-cultural rehabilitation: An international perspective. 1-7. London: W.B. Sounders.

Nosek, P. (2004). *Secondary Conditions among Women with Disabilities.* Center for Research on Women with Disabilities (CROWD) Baylor College of Medicine, Houston, TX.

Patrick, D. L. (1997). Rethinking prevention for people with disabilities: a conceptual model for promoting health. *American Journal of Health Promotion*, 11: 257-260.

Riddley, C. R., Mendosa, D. W., Kanitz, B. E. Angermeier, L. & Zenk, R. (1994). Cultural sensitivity in multicultural counseling: A perceptual schema. *Journal of Counseling Psychology*, 41, 125-136.

Rimmer, J. H. (1999). Health promotion for people with disabilities: The emerging paradigm shift from disability prevention to prevention of secondary conditions. *Journal of Physical Therapy*, 79, 495-502.

Stone, J. H. (2005). Culture and Disability: Providing culturally competent services. Multicultural aspects of counseling series 21. Thousand Oaks, CA: Sage Publications.

Sue, D. W., Arrendondo, P. & McDavis, R. J. (1992). Multicultural counseling competencies and standards: A call to the profession. *Journal of Multicultural Counseling and Development*, 20, 64-88.

U. S. Department of Health and Human Services. (2005). *The Surgeon General's Call to Action: To Improve the Health and Wellness of Persons with Disabilities.* Office of the Surgeon General, Washington DC.

Ware, N. C. & Kleinman (1992). Culture and somatic experience: The social course of illness in Neurasthenoa and Chronic Fatigue Syndrome. *Psychosomatic Medicine*, 54: 546-560.

Wong-Hernandez, L. & Wong, D. W. (2002). The effects of language and culture variables to the rehabilitation of bilingual and bicultural consumers: A review of literature study focusing on Hispanic Americans and Asian Americans. *Disability Studies Quarterly*, 22(2), 109-127.

Wong, D.W., & Wong- Hernandez, L. (November, 2007). Serving Individuals with Disabilities from Diverse Culture and Ethnic Backgrounds—Part 1. Retrieved February 3, 2008, from TIRR (The Institute for Rehabilitation and Research *http://www.tirr. org/*).

Wong, D.W., & Wong- Hernandez, L. (November, 2007). Serving Individuals with Disabilities from Diverse Culture and Ethnic Backgrounds—Part 2. Retrieved February 3, 2008, from TIRR (The Institute for Rehabilitation and Research *http://www.tirr. org/*).

4

The Changing American Family: The View from Social Texts

E. Doyle McCarthy
Sandra Farganis

Abstract

Changes in American families since the mid-twentieth century are described with special attention given to the dissemination of these views of families by the social sciences, especially sociology. The popularization of the ideas about marriage, child-rearing, and family life coming from both sociology and psychology has contributed to cultural changes in American life and collective behavior, particularly the new idea and image of the "diversity" of family forms and "changing families." The social and psychological sciences have not acted as independent forces for change; they simultaneously reflect and contribute to the changes they study and describe. While the primary functions of the social sciences have been to offer objective and unsentimental views of the family as a "social institution" among other social institutions, their rational and secular perspectives have had an impact—largely unintentional—on everyday life and contemporary culture. The value of family sociology is discussed. Proposals for a public family sociology are outlined—a sociology accessible to an educated lay public and to family practitioners and therapists.

Today's American family is about a half century old, although its roots have been traced to social and economic changes of the early twentieth century. Its immediate social location is American society after World War II, a world variously labeled "the welfare state," "the new industrial state," the "post-industrial society," or "postmodernity." Social scientists have chronicled the U.S. family's development over a five- or six-decade period (from the 1940s to today), a time of unprecedented change in the forms of industry, work, technology, and the values of America's people.

In an earlier paper (McCarthy, 1983), it was argued that the contemporary American family is a creation of contemporary social science. By this, we mean that the findings of the extensive investigations of the social science community were disseminated, largely through mass media and political policy-making, and that this process transmuted social scientific conceptual reality into common coin of the realm. Our intention in this chapter is to present that conceptual reality in its various forms and manifestations: we shall describe the ways the American family has been typically portrayed by social scientists, largely through some of the leading textbooks in family sociology. In this chapter we will be using the singular "the family" to discuss recent changes in this social institution (cf. Cherlin 2008a, pp. 30-31), particularly the ways that sociologists have recently studied and portrayed the family. This usage does not overlook the many forms that family life has taken in recent decades. Rather, its intention is to emphasize its collective and institutional forms and functions in American life today. However different the forms that families have taken in recent decades, sociology's perspective contributes to an understanding of how the lived experiences of men, women, and children in families today share important features. The institution of the family is best understood as both a *response* to shared structural features of today's economy and culture, as well as an institution that is itself a *force facilitating change* still further (Berger, 2002, chap. 4).

Sociological and psychological discourse occupies a special place in modern societies like our own. As modern disciplines, they developed as systematic attempts to describe the social and mental worlds of modernity. For this reason, their perspectives on various aspects of social reality, like the family, are characterized by types of thinking, which came about only in the last two hundred years or so of human history. Modern disciplines, like sociology, developed in response to both changes in the forms of social life and their increasing complexification. At the same time, sociology served to change and rationalize that world still further, as its practitioners made their way into those institutions, which fostered and distributed its knowledge: the academy, the government, public policy centers, public and private foundations, and welfare agencies. Thus, sociological discourse occupies a special place on the modern scene: it emerges to inquire into the nature of modernity and its institutions while at the same time fostering a rational perspective on social practices and institutions. Stated simply, our main thesis is that sociology describes and is itself an element of its description. Sociology affects changes in the institutions it investigates (Gans, 1989; Farganis, 1996; McCarthy, 1996).

With respect to the contemporary family, sociology, by its own account, sets about the task of describing and interpreting the various ways the family has changed during the last century and, most especially, since the 1940s. One important result of the development of the sociology of the family is its role in awakening people's interests in family-related concerns: sexuality, marriage, child-rearing. More specifically, sociology plays a central role in communicating the image of the contemporary family in crisis and change. In the words of Margaret Mead, whose anthropological works have played a special role in relativizing people's images of the family: "The American family is at the center of American concern at the present time; its strengths and weaknesses, its past and its future are being subjected to every kind of scrutiny, pessimistic and optimistic" (1959, p. 116). Mead suggests that because of the attention paid to the family by sociology, people's concerns about the family gave birth to both critics and supporters—those who would announce the "end of the family" and those who would argue that the family was "here to stay." We would argue that in both cases there is clearly an awareness of new *models or forms* of family and family life, that these changes have given rise to a greater public scrutiny of American families, and that many of the changes of recent decades have also occasioned the "family wars" (Berger & Berger, 1983) or "family politics" (Dionne, 1991).

We are not arguing that sociology single-handedly creates change, but that sociological description and discourse are cultural forms promulgating change of a particular kind. The development of social science takes place against the backdrop of a broader social context of change, known under the social scientific term—one with its own history of academic controversies—"modernization." Modern disciplines like the social and psychological sciences both reflected those changes and promulgated them. Accordingly, sociology fosters its own rationalizing vision of social reality both in its proclivity for fact-gathering and in its attempt to detach itself from the objects of its inquiries. In this way, sociology fosters modes of thinking about marriage and family life that bear an uneasy relation to traditional, moral, and religious perspectives on the nature of sexuality, marriage, and child-rearing. These sociological modes of thinking are grounded in science, are analytical and empirically-based, and are value-free in intent (Cherlin 2008a, pp. 16-21). Thus, in its truest sense, the import of sociological inquiry is its antagonism to myth. In stating things in this way, we are not so much celebrating sociology's undermining of commonly held ideas and ideas about families; rather, we are pointing to one important function of sociological description: it offers a "debunking" view of all social institutions (Berger, 1963, chap. 2). In the process of describing the facts at hand (about marriage, divorce, family life, childrearing), sociologists are intent on uncovering the *social sources of our beliefs about what we do*—including the various ways Americans actually live, how they think, and what they have to say about, for example, marriage, divorce, abortion, gay marriage, to name a few of the current issues on our (collective) minds today.

Sociology's antagonism to "myths" about families is a theme in some of sociology's leading family textbooks and authors today. To summarize these arguments: the empirical study of today's families contributes to an undermining of leading "myths" about family life—the end of the extended family, the notion that "opposites attract," or that people marry for love—and it is important for us, these authors argue, to recognize that certain common beliefs are wrong (Lauer & Lauer, 2007; Aulette, 2007; Zinn & Eitzen, 2005). This theme was also the theme of a book by family historian, Stephanie Coontz, *The Way We Never Were* (1992). Studying family history enables us, she argues, to dispel the many myths we have about American families, separating nostalgic and ideological conceptions about family from the realities of family life then and now (see also Coontz, 1997; 2005; Ahrons, 2007).

The related theme of *changing families* is, perhaps, the centerpiece of sociology textbooks and studies. For Coontz, the historian, the changes in marriage and family life are traced to the development of modern industrial society. For sociologists, the focus is more immediate—"the fundamental ways in which the family as a social institution has changed over the past half century" (Cherlin, 2008a, p. 503). Families today, most family sociologists tell us, are very different from what they used to be. Families vary across time and within societies (Zinn & Eitzen, 2005; Lauer & Lauer, 2007; Ferguson, 2007; Cherlin, 2008a). But the clearest and most consistent message from family sociologists today is that American families have undergone major changes in the closing decades of the twentieth century (Furstenberg, 2008; Morgan, 1996; Wetzel, 1990), a topic we will return to below.

Family Sociology and Social Change

Sociological inquiry has often developed in response to social changes and family sociology is no exception. From its beginnings in the period 1890-1930, sociology's classical works represented a response to the dramatic political, economic, and social events and changes that took place in eighteenth- and nineteenth-century Europe. As Robert Nisbet (1976) has argued, in the writings of Emile Durkheim, Max Weber, and Georg Simmel we find a strong sense of ambivalence about the changes they were witnessing, changes understood by many of their contemporaries as indications of progress. Similarly, the changes in family life recorded by sociologists today, draw a variety of responses from sociologists themselves as well as the public, revealing high levels of political involvement in these changes, as well as high levels of public anxiety about the changes facing families and children today (Skolnick, 1991). In fact, the field of family therapy itself can be seen as a response to today's changes in families and in the meanings of parenting, marriage, gender, and sexuality.

As many have indicated, almost all of the changes families face today can be traced to changes associated with industrialization in its various phases. In fact, family sociology's origins began in America in the late nineteenth century, coinciding with changes in both marriage and family life, especially industrialization and urbanization; the empirical study of the family was part of the rise of sociology in America in that period (e.g., Small & Vincent, 1894). Decades later, the developing field of social psychology provided a second framework within which to study the socializing effects of family relationships (e.g., Karpf, 1932). Within these two fields—urban sociology and social psychology—social scientists described the changes wrought on family life and relations by urbanization, immigrant culture, poverty, and social change.

In its initial stages in the early twentieth century, principally in the writings of sociologists at Columbia University and the University of Chicago, family sociology was closely aligned with social reform and social welfare. This approach found expression in the need to solve the problems imposed on the family by social change and to strengthen it against the forces of modernization and urbanization. Later, the history of family sociology, from the late 1920s to the present day, was characterized by two seemingly disparate tendencies: on the one hand, sociology's disengagement from reformist concerns and its pursuit of an empirical study of family life; on the other hand, its developing association with the area of public policy studies. In fact, the uses of sociology for social policy has continued and grown almost uninterrupted since this early period.

Particularly since the Carter administration in the 1970s, family policy studies comprise the largest portion of studies and publications on the family. These studies include works on human sexuality, abortion, women's rights, domestic violence, the aged, the rearing and education of children, and alternative forms of marriage. Each of these issues bears on the current perception of the contemporary American family as an institution that is either in "crisis" and/or undergoing rapid and inevitable "change." For example, efforts to outline a national family policy or to offer piecemeal reforms can be seen as a response to what some believe to be a crisis in America's families of extraordinary proportion—a crisis which has called for intensive governmental intervention in family life. Developments like these have generated a critical sociological literature (e.g., Lasch, 1977; Steiner, 1981; Berger & Berger, 1983; Berger, 2002). A context of social change has provided the impetus for family sociology from its inception, in the period of urban growth between both world wars, right up to the present day. At the same time, the empirical study of family life has expanded with the added impetus of government sponsored research and the growing conviction that government bears a responsibility toward the family as an institution. Besides government support of family studies, two factors are critical in the expansion and application of family sociology: first, the unprecedented growth of family-related professions in the post-World War II years (counseling and therapy, social work, education, medicine and health); second, the demographic changes of this same period. These two developments are clearly interrelated.

Demographic Changes of the Post-War Years

What were the types of changes that were studied and recorded by sociologists? In many ways, they were demographic changes (in births, deaths, and longevity) occurring first in the late nineteenth and early twentieth centuries when family life was shaped by America's increasing immigrant populations and the simultaneous growth in America's cities. However, in the post-World War II period, the demographic changes were, in large part, brought about by the "baby boom," referring to those born in the U.S. from 1946 to 1964 (Wetzel, 1990) and to the changes that occurred during the lifespan of this baby boom generation. Social scientists identified the baby boom itself as a force in many of the economic, geographic, and social changes of that time, leading to major governmental agencies and policies in education, health care, housing, work, and social welfare. In the words of two family sociologists: "Perhaps no event during the twentieth century will have as far-reaching consequences for American society as the post-World War II baby boom" (Masnick & Bane, 1980).

In the period of the baby boom of the late 1940s and 1950s, more than 42 million babies were born in the United States, more than 4.2 million a year. This is about twice the number born to the generation of adults raising families in the 1930s. Since 1961 the number has declined, reaching a low of 3.1 million births in 1975. The total has remained between 3.1 and 3.4 million a year ever since (Masnick & Bane, 1980). Since the early 1970s, the birth rate has been below "replacement level," meaning that if the rate continued at that level over time, the population would decline. Of course, the factors countering such an effect would be death rates and immigration rates. While birth rates today are higher among the poor and racial and ethnic minorities than among non-poor whites, the declines in birth rates occurred in all racial, ethnic, and class groupings. In keeping with these figures, sociologists have observed changes over time in the ideal number of children for families, with changing preferences for smaller families reflected in declining birth rates over time (Lauer & Lauer, 2007, pp. 274-75).

Birthrates and changes in family size, have, of course, been studied relative to women's increased presence in the workforce over this period, an issue that has received a great deal of attention in textbooks (Aulette, 2007, chap. 6; Ferguson, 2007, part X; Zinn & Eitzen, 2005, chap. 5; Lauer & Lauer, 2007, chap. 12). In fact, this topic—work and home—is typically given an entire chapter in the texts we reviewed, raising further questions about its place of prominence in the textbook literature. Is it due to the political and social issues surrounding working mothers? If so, why? Is it principally the unresolved questions—political as well as personal— about childcare when almost three quarters of mothers of young children are in the labor force? Brigitte Berger's treatment (2002, pp. 192-204) of the issue, insists that we distinguish the *separate issues involved with "women and work"*: gender equality in the workplace, women's interests (in working inside or outside the home), and child development. These three issues are not the same and they raise separate issues and concerns about women, women's rights, children, and childcare.

The theme of "work and home" points to one of the most important changes for families today, at least if we use the textbooks as an indicator. In the early twentieth century few married women worked outside the home, about one in five (20 percent). By 1960, fewer that one third (30 percent) were in the labor force; by 1990 this proportion had almost doubled; today about half of women (from ages sixteen and older) are working outside the home (Hutter, 1998, p. 335; Lauer & Lauer, 2007, pp. 250-51; Aulette, 2007, pp. 140-41). These changes in women working have taken place among all class, racial, and ethnic groupings, so that growing numbers of women from all of these groups combine mother-hood with paid employment, even when their children are young (Spain and Bianchi 1996). The increase of women in the workforce is described by family sociologist, Andrew Cherlin (2008a, p. 261) as a major and significant social movement with important outcomes: "This great move-ment of married women into the labor force is one of the most important changes in American family life in the past century. It has profoundly altered women's and men's lives." Returning to the subject of the baby boom of the 1940s and 1950s—the highest fertility rate in the twentieth century—the women born during this period (1940s-1950s) were the first generation to enter the workforce in such high proportions, relative to their mothers and grandmothers.

The baby boom generation (with ages ranging today from the early for-ties to age sixty) are those who have already had an impact on American life and its families by virtue of their numbers and lifestyles. Studies from census and population reports provide the following profiles of them: they are better educated than the generations before them; their women have entered the work force in larger numbers; they have left home at a younger age than their predecessors and, as unmarried people, have set up households alone or with other young people. This generation delayed marriage longer (partly due to their extended years of schooling) and, in comparison with other generations, they have higher proportions of those who are divorced or who have never married (at comparable ages) (Coontz, 2005, chap. 13; Casper and Bianchi, 2008).

It was predicted that as many as 40 percent of women born in the 1950s, for example, remained childless or had only one child during their lifetimes. These factors are related to a number of changes: the increasing number of women who will spend a relatively short period of their lives child-bearing and child-raising (due to birth control, abortion, work, and their own longevity); increases in childless marriages; a continued rise in the employment of women outside the home. If one also considers the rise in single-parent households, due to rising divorce rates and the number of unmarried people, *demographers accurately predicted from the decade of the 1980s and after, an increase in the number of two-worker families, an increase in single-parent families resulting from divorce, an increase in one-child or childless marriages, and a continued trend toward households of the unmarried living alone or with others.*

Many of these social facts are familiar to us, since they are communi-cated to us by social scientists, journalists, and politicians. However, it is also useful to place some of these observations within the framework of larger historical and demographic trends. In this way their impact is not so much changed but, perhaps, better understood. By way of illustration, we consider declining fertility rates and the reported rise of single-parent households. Here, the analyses of Masnick and Bane (1980) are particularly useful (cf. Wetzel, 1990; Furstenberg, 2007).

They report that far from being abnormal, the lower rates of fertility and marriage of young adults today are consistent with long-term trends. Since until the 1940s, fertility rates had been consistently declining, marriage rates had begun to level off, and divorce rates were consistently rising. Only in the case of the generation born between 1920 and 1940 were fertility rates higher and divorce rates lower. In the authors' words: "Had the 1940s and 1950s not happened, today's young adults would appear to be behaving normally.... However, when the benchmark chosen to judge the family patterns of today's young adults is that of their parents' generation, those born since 1940 do appear deviant" (Masnick & Bane, 1980, pp. 2-3).

It is also useful to put the reported numbers of families headed by women in perspective. Trends since 1950 clearly indicate a rise in the proportion of families made up of women living with children or other relatives (not husbands). In the same period there has also been a decline in the proportion of husband/wife households in relation to all households. However, the broader trend shows 1940 to have had an equally high percentage of families headed by women (15.1 percent in 1940; 14.4 percent in 1978). In 1940 and earlier, a woman who headed a family was much more likely to be a middle-aged widow living with her children or an older woman living with adult children or a sibling of hers (Uhlenberg, 1980). Since 1978, women heads-of-households more typically reflected the fact that there were a higher number of divorced or separated women in the population (Masnick & Bane, 1980; cf. Bane, 1976, chap. 8; Coontz, 1992, chap. 9).

Furthermore, the rising divorce rates of the last few decades do not mean that fewer children now live with their parents than in earlier generations. As Bane reported in her 1976 study, the proportion of children who live with *at least one of their parents* rather than with relatives, with foster parents, or in institutions has been steadily rising during the last decades of the twentieth century. This is in large part due to declining death rates of adults as well as the increasing numbers of widowed and divorced women who continued living with their children after their marriage ended. Overall, the declining death rates counteracted the rising divorce rates in the period from about 1930 to 1960. Only for children born in the early 1960s did rising divorce rates begin to counteract the effect of falling death rates. In Bane's words: "The proportion of children who experienced a parental disruption fell until then; only recently has disruption increased" (1976, pp. 12-13; cf. Coontz, 1992, pp. 221-225).

As we have tried to show by these few examples, a look at the historical trends provides a more complete and accurate picture of recent changes in the American family. However, even when some of these trends, say, in household composition and divorce rates, are considered, the American family has clearly undergone major changes in recent decades—changes that form the central arguments of the textbooks. Not only has "the family" (the cultural and "traditional" ideal discussed above) been replaced by an acceptance of more varied institutional forms—"families" or "diversity" in families, but there is evidence that the *meanings* associated with marriage and family life have also changed remarkably. Again, the demographic changes in this movement are important, if not the principal source or cause of these changes. Along with Cherlin (2008a), we are pointing especially to the changes brought about by women in the work force, but also to increased divorce rates, decreasing birthrates, and the increase in men and women who "never marry."

From the perspective of family studies, the changes that occurred in U.S. families in the last decades of the twentieth century have been truly remarkable, representing a "major shift...in the form and function" of the family (Furstenberg, 2008, p. 359; cf. Cherlin 2004). These include changes *in people's behaviors* (with respect to marrying, divorcing, remarrying, parenting), *in the increasingly diverse types of households* (one- or two-parent households, same-sex or opposite-sex parents, natural and adoptive parents, families with children and stepchildren), and changes *in the ways people think about and evaluate the institutions of marriage and family*—changes in the cultures people draw from and use in their own lives and how they evaluate others' lives. These changes have taken many forms.

The changes consistently identified by both social scientists and historians include: the decline, relative to mid-twentieth century, in the exclusive role of woman-as-homemaker and the movement of women into the labor force. These two facts are clearly related, although in complex ways, to rising divorce rates, single-parent households, and to changing relations of couples with respect to the meanings of marriage, sex, and gender roles. These changes—so important to our understanding of family change—also point to a more general movement of Americans away from the *authority* of both men (husband/father) and parents (both men and women) to a more democratic or egalitarian ("individualist") marriage and family structure, what Anthony Giddens (1992) has described as a "democratization of the personal sphere," a greater elaboration of individuality in intimate relations and in marriage and family life. In many important ways, *the change from "the family" to "families," from a single standard of marriage and family life to a recognition and acceptance by many of diversity in marriage and family life, is part of a number of cultural changes in American life today that include rising expectations about intimacy and sexuality, together with a sense of "choice" in matters of sexual identity, marriage, divorce, and parenting* (Coontz, 2005, chap. 16; Cherlin, 2008a, chap. 15; Cancian, 1987, chap. 3). Marriage, to take one important example, is increasingly viewed as a matter of one's own choice, a feature of one's self-identity, and a means of self-fulfillment. In sociological terms this means that marriage is no longer seen as an *institution* as much as a "relationship" between equal partners seeking intimacy and fulfillment. Similarly, the willingness of most Americans to accept the rights of others to live their own lives—including those with whom they might disagree on issues of sex, marriage, and family—reflects the relatively new and widespread idea that marriage and family life is about "choice"—freely chosen arrangements for living (Cherlin, 2008a, p. 502; cf. Cherlin, 1999). Put differently, over the last half century, marriage and family have become increasingly viewed as *human* enterprises or creations, albeit with important symbolic and individual value, but no longer as social and religious *facticities* that encompass people's lives. Today, we are witnessing the expansion of "personal choice" in matters of sex, sexual identity, marriage, and parenting, a cultural trend already identified by social scientists for some time (Coontz, 2007; McClay, 1994; Bellah et al, 1985; Riesman, 1950).

These are the pressing issues of American families today reflected in many of the family texts. The meanings people give to "marriage" and "family" today—individual, personal, emotional—also provide a context for understanding the phenomenon of "diversity" itself, a theme so central to the sociology textbooks. For the value of personal "choice," extended to the domain of marriage and family life, has acted as a catalyst producing even more diversity and tolerance of diversity in American life, just as it has been the source of "family wars" in politics. According to Cherlin (2008a, p. 502; cf. Cherlin, 1999), Americans "may value the traditional family, but they accept family diversity as inevitable, and perhaps beneficial." "Many people," he concludes, "accept the fact that for better or worse, we live in an era with a variety of family forms, including cohabiting unions, dual-earner married couples, breadwinner-homemaker couples, single-parent families, step-families, and same-sex marriages and domestic partnerships."

The image of the family that can be drawn from these descriptions and trends—an image studied and communicated to the American public—is one that is at odds with what has been considered to have been the ideal of the "traditional" nuclear American family which, oddly enough, is associated solely with the post-World War II period in U.S. history. This ideal image—born of America's Cold War era and its ethos of emotional and familial containment—included a breadwinner husband and home-maker wife and their children, living in a climate of relative affluence and comfort in a suburban or small town home (May, 1999; Oakes, 1994, chap. 4). Today's diverse family image is also at odds with the lifestyles of the generation of Americans born between 1920 and 1940, today ages sixty-seven to eighty-seven. For that generation probably achieved the traditional ideal more than earlier generations, many of whom lived in periods of war or economic hardship, who lived and worked as immigrants in America's burgeoning cities or its then dominant rural areas (Coontz, 1992, chap. 1; Furstenberg, 2007; Wetzel, 1990).

As to the current generations of America's young adults and those just approaching middle age, not only have their economic expectations altered, but so have their images and ideals of sex, marriage, and family life. If the textbooks are a register of changes, the idea of "diversity" in these trends and living arrangements has characterized American life and politics in recent decades. As we have argued, sociology has clearly had a role in shaping Americans' consciousness of our families and our ideals of families. This collective awareness of the plurality of household arrange-ments, of the diversity of family and marriage forms that characterize most Americans today, includes: two-worker households; middle-aged couples whose children moved away; childless couples; the unmarried with children; retired couples; single-parent families; gay, lesbian, and transgender couples; and immigrant and transnational families. According to the textbooks, *a pluralistic family form has impressed itself as a new image on the contemporary consciousness of Americans*. And, however much that image draws various moral and political responses, it seems to have gained legitimacy among a large number of Americans, while "the family" has been increasingly delegitimated (Stacey, 1993), and while marriage is undergoing "deinstitutionalization" (Cherlin, 2004). Among other things, this means that marriage has lost its once-dominant role in the regulation of sex and the raising of children. This has also been accompanied by the ability of many to live their lives outside of marriage without either legal or social disadvantages. In many ways, this development—marriage's deinstitutionalization—is part of today's family "diversity." It is a change far reaching in its social consequences.

Social Science as Impetus for Change

What are the implications of these changes and of people's collective consciousness of them? Some have observed that since the decade of the 1960s, America has passed through periods of substantive change in political values, in the range and depth of their religious commitments, in the role of religion in political life, and in other social ideas and ideals, particularly as these bear on sex and marriage, family life, and child rearing (Bell, 1996; Bellah, Madsen, Sullivan, & Swidler, 1985; Putnam, 2000; Wuthnow, 1998). While no one has suggested that these changes have occurred uniformly for all groups, classes, regions, and communities, certain generalizations about Americans in the last half century indicate a climate of change in people's perceptions of themselves, their work, and family life (Veroff, Kulka, & Douvan, 1981; Veroff, Douvan, & Kulka, 1981). This brings us back to the central arguments of this chapter: *the contemporary role of social science in both reflecting and in bringing about a certain type of cultural change in American life today.*

In particular, the period of change from the 1950s to the present coincided with the growing importance of social scientific research in government, business, and universities. Benefiting from the post-World War II economic boom, sociology received its research funds from government agencies, private foundations, and business organizations. These changes continue unabated to the present time. In some senses, we can say that the role of the social sciences in American life and culture has grown with each decade. With a number of different types of supports from the public and the private sector, sociologists have moved into new fields of specialization: military, medical, and industrial sociology, communications, public opinion, criminology, and marriage and family therapy and counseling, to name but a few. Similarly, empirical research has gained considerable status both within the profession and in other disciplines, achieving the status of a prestigious and financially-supported professional activity.

During the same period, the value and the social role of U.S. sociologists have been judged by our *social utility.* In the textbooks of the 1940s and 1950s for example, a central theme is that of the sociologist as a pragmatist and practitioner whose knowledge can be used to solve immediate practical problems. Sociology is seen as a field of inquiry capable of providing practical answers to a variety of social problems. Sociological knowledge "will be of use no matter what the occupation," William F. Ogburn wrote in 1940. Students of sociology "will be ... prepared to direct the social changes ahead" (Ogburn & Nimkoff, 1940; cf. Williams, 1951; Rumney & Maier, 1953; Rose, 1956). Similarly, in a leading 1958 text, the role of the sociologist engaged in administrative research is discussed; the sociologist solves concrete problems and can advise others about the proper means for achieving practical goals, winning an election, gaining support for a public policy, avoiding crises such as strikes (Landis, 1958, p. xix).

In his 1964 *Handbook of Marriage and the Family,* Harold Christensen (1964, pp. 3-32) states that during the same decades, the field of family sociology had gained respect and there had been an increasing acceptance of its scientific viewpoint. Substantive reports and empirical studies were being disseminated and the National Council on Family Relations had been formed. Its official publications were the *Journal of Marriage and the Family* and *The Family Coordinator.* As in the field of sociology, family research was problem-oriented and reflected people's growing concerns for marital and family stability and child-rearing. As noted in the 1977 issue of *Daedalus* on the family (p. ix), "In family studies, the line between theory and practice—between the theoretical and the applied—is not nearly so fixed as it is in certain other areas. If home economics is theoretical, it also has immediate implications for practice; the same may be said for much of the work that is proceeding in disciplines as various as psychology, history, anthropology, and sociology."

In the influential family textbook by Zinn and Eitzen (2005), first published in 1985, we find an example of this prevailing view *that the study of the family needs to be both empirically grounded and socially useful.* To highlight the authors' arguments: (1) the purpose of the text is to demythologize the family by examining its many actual forms and functions; (2) the important variables for study are class, race, gender, and sexuality; (3) one should put aside a theory of the family (structural-functionalism) that assumes an ideal-typical nuclear family and replace it with a historical-empirical account of "structural-diversity" (2005, p. xii); (5) family forms and functions are not changed by values, but by social and economic particulars.

The authors argue that the acknowledged changes in families in recent decades point to a "paradigm shift" in family studies, one which they value, a "dramatic period of diversification in family studies" that includes a "greater diversity in domestic life," a freeing of women and men from conventional marriages, and new family and household arrangements (p. 436). In place of the contested idea of "the family;" today, they argue, we have a pluralism of forms; "family boundaries are becoming more ambiguous" (p.478). As this summary makes clear, the text is clearly progressive in its affirmation of the family as a social and historical construct (p. 479). The contribution of the social sciences is to develop policies that provide "safety nets" for that plurality of family forms to exist.

As can be seen from this summary of some of the earlier and contemporary textbooks, the link between sociology and applied fields (family and child therapy, mental health and counseling, social work) has continued to develop over time: sociology can be of use to practitioners just as practitioners can test the findings and interpretations of the social scientists. In fact, the growing alliance between sociology and family practitioners, from the 1920s to today, can be considered one of the main conduits carrying sociological knowledge into the household itself. It is of this alliance that Christopher Lasch (1977, chaps. 5 & 8) wrote about so critically, arguing that the contemporary family is invaded by family practitioners whose efforts on its behalf undermine its continued existence. The family struggles to conform to an ideal imposed on it from without. This ideal reflects the perspectives of the social and psychological sciences, both of which gained recognition and authority during the decades following the war. Lasch identifies several features of the family practitioner approach. These include the therapeutic values of tolerance, personal growth, and psychic maturity, and the extolling of companionship, self-realization, and happiness over authority, loyalty, and obligation.

The influence of social science on family life is also felt in ways that are more indirect but, perhaps, even more far-reaching. Here, we can speak of an *ethos* created by the dissemination of knowledges by the social and psychological sciences—an ethos that has itself become part of American culture, just as it has drawn from that culture's individualist, pragmatic, and utilitarian dimensions. For example, during the period from the 1950s to the 1970s, American society underwent what could be called a social and psychological revolution, a shift toward a decidedly more psychological orientation in our culture. According to some critics, this change coincided with the growth of a "new class" of upwardly mobile, college-educated individuals who parented the baby boom generation—a class more liberal, intellectual, and secular than members of America's traditional middle classes (Bensman & Vidich, 1971; Vidich & Bensman, 1958). This class, in its various social and regional groupings, acted as carriers of a culture that set itself against America's (small town) middle class and its (Protestant) religion and morality. In its place the social and psychological sciences provided a perspective that was both more humanistic and secular. These modern disciplines can be said to have provided an ethos within which the contemporary family developed. As one observer notes, in contrast to the traditional image of the family, the contemporary family "is no longer seen as a compensatory institution, but as a community whose end is the support, the fulfillment, and the health and satisfaction of its individual members. The family no longer serves mainly to nurture the citizen, the religious person, or even the economic person. It is there to serve psychological man" (Orr, 1980, p. 380).

While these arguments on the role of psychology and therapy in American culture and family life are clearly valid today (Illouz, 2007) and deserve sociological study and critique, the relationship of sociology to American culture and life is remarkably more varied in the way sociology sees itself vis-à-vis American society. For example, today we are witnessing movements in sociology that would revitalize a publicly-engaged sociology (Mills, 1959; Jacoby, 1987; Gans, 1989; Burawoy, 2005), one that would complement professional sociology. Michael Burawoy's, "For Public Sociology," his 2004 presidential address, proposes "a back-translation, taking knowledge back to those from whom it came, making public issues out of private troubles, and thus regenerating sociology's moral fiber" (2005, p. 5). In an earlier presidential address, the sociologist Herbert Gans (1989) introduced the concept "public sociologists" as those who report their work to an educated lay public in an accessible written form; a sociology that reveals a broad grasp of American culture and institutions; a sociology that offers both commentary and social criticism (p. 7).

Public Family Sociology

In pointing to these proposals by Gans and Burawoy, we want to consider the implications of a public sociology for family practitioners. As we have outlined here, the historical relationship of sociology to the applied fields of family policy and family therapy has been one where practitioners and sociologists work together—albeit with relatively distinct roles and functions—to address issues like poverty, aging parents, childcare, physical and mental illness and treatment—a sociological model based on the twin ideas of (first) the value of the *usefulness* of sociology for addressing social problems, and (second) the idea that sociology's principal contribution to families and family practitioners is its empirically-based knowledge about families—portraits of family life, the choices they make, their own spoken "values" and "attitudes." In light of the recent statements by Gans and Burawoy, which we endorse, we think that these longstanding sociological models can benefit from an overhaul. For while we endorse the *value* of empiricism for sociology and its publics, we also subscribe to a public sociology whose principal interest is in making sociological knowledge accessible to an educated lay public as well as to family professionals and paraprofessionals.

Public family sociology could address a number of topics relatively untouched by sociologists today and, more typically, addressed by journalists and essayists: a sociology-of-knowledge account of the current debates about families and family policy, one characterized by a self-critical and reflexive dimension. A second topic—a service to the public and to sociology itself—could be a debunking examination of popular sociology that sorts out the good and bad versions of this genre, based on informed readings of the sociology of the family (Gans, 1989, pp. 7-9). Public sociology brings sociology back to its tradition of *social criticism.*

In this chapter, we have examined—using sociological presuppositions—some of our own discipline's textbooks with a view toward understanding some of the ways that the textbooks operate in the culture at large: how textbook writers, using empirical studies of families, provide both *knowledge of* and *images of* American families today; how, for example, these knowledges and images operate not merely as "facts learned," but also as sources for changes in how people think about families (and themselves) and, by extension, how family practitioners think about the families to whom they provide services. Our own project, whatever its social value, clearly does *not* constitute a social critique of the textbooks we studied. But we conclude by pointing our readers in that direction. Such an enterprise would be an example of the type of public sociology discussed here. For it would engage and evaluate sociologists themselves as participants in the current discussions and debates about the family today. A socially-critical sociology also asks the questions—held suspect today for their moralism—What is a good society? What is sociology's role in bringing it about (Gans, 1989, p. 5)?

Finally, a critical family sociology might address the issue highlighted in one leading family textbook (Cherlin, 2008a, pp. 505-512) of "personal life" in late modern societies. The shape of individualism (also, personalism and emotivism) in twenty-first-century America is already an important subject addressed within sociological discourse (Bellah et al, 1985; Bell, 1996; Giddens, 1991; 1992). Its consequences have grown as we witness the transformation of the *social meanings* of marriage and family life from communal and community institutions to individual-based ones where the prevailing discourse is choice-based, therapeutic, personalistic, and emotivist. The idea that "the personal is political" is an idea that originated in American feminist theory of the 1960s (Zaretsky, 1986). The phrase means that people's experiences and feelings are not so much "their own" as they are shaped and limited in important ways by the "social" and "political." To understand "the personal is political" is to engage the sociological imagination (Mills, 1959). It questions the social relations and structures, the prevailing images and attitudes and feelings surrounding "the family" and our commitment to its importance for ourselves and our society. It asks whether and which families can and should be self-sufficient, whether (and on what grounds) marriage should be confined to couples of the opposite sex, whether caring for our children is a private or public good. These are only some of the questions that a critical sociology might address. Its value as "public sociology" rests on its empirical base, its accessible prose and style of address, its broad and social purview; its subject matter is both deeply felt and consequential for many. This is the promise and challenge of public sociology (Burawoy, 2005, p. 5).

References

Ahrons, C. (2007). No easy answers: Why the popular view of divorce is wrong. In S. J. Ferguson (Ed.), *Shifting the Center: Understanding Contemporary Families* (3rd ed.), (pp. 523-534). New York: McGraw-Hill.

Aulette, J. R. (2007). *Changing American Families* (2nd ed.). Boston: Allyn & Bacon.

Bane, M. J. (1976). *Here to Stay: American Families in the Twentieth Century.* New York: Basic Books.

Bell, D. (1973). *The Coming of Post-Industrial Society.* New York: Basic Books.

Bell, D. (1996). *The Cultural Contradictions of Capitalism* (20th anniversary ed.). New York: Basic Books.

Bellah, R., Madsen R., Sullivan, W. M., & Swidler, A. (1985). *Habits of the Heart: Individualism and Commitment in American Life.* Berkeley, CA: University of California Press.

Bensman, J. & Vidich, A. J. (1971). *The New American Society.* New York: Quadrangle Books.

Berger, B. (2002). *The Family in the Modern Age: More Than a Lifestyle Choice.* New Brunswick, NJ: Transaction Publishers.

Berger, B. & Berger, P. L. (1983). *The War over the Family: Capturing the Middle Ground.* New York: Double Day/Anchor.

Berger, P.L. (1963). *Invitation to Sociology.* New York: Doubleday.

Berger, P.L. (1967). *The Sacred Canopy.* New York: Doubleday.

Berger, P. L., Berger, B., & Hansfried, K. (1973). *The Homeless Mind.* New York: Random House.

Burawoy, M. (2005). For public sociologies. 2004 Presidential address, American Sociological Association. *American Sociological Review* 70 (1), pp. 4-28.

Cancian, F. M. (1987). *Love in America: Gender and self-development.* New York: Cambridge University Press.

Casper, L. & Bianchi, S. M. (2002/2008). A "quieting" of family change. In A. J. Cherlin (Ed.) *Public and Private Families: A Reader* 5/e, (pp. 3-28). New York: McGraw-Hill.

Cherlin, A.J. (1999). "I'm O.K., you're selfish." *The New York Times Magazine,* pp. 44-46.

Cherlin, A.J. (2004). The deinstitutionalization of marriage. *Journal of Marriage and the Family,* 66 (November), pp. 848-861.

Cherlin, A.J. (2008a). *Public and Private Families: An Introduction* (5th ed.). New York: McGraw-Hill.

Cherlin, A.J. (Ed.) (2008b). *Public and Private Families: A Reader (5th ed.).* New York: McGraw-Hill.

Christensen, H.T. (Ed.). (1964). *Handbook of Marriage and the Family.* Chicago: Rand McNally.

Coontz, S. (1997). *The Way We Really Are: Coming to Terms with America's Changing Families.* New York: Basic Books.

Coontz, S. (1992). *The Way We Never Were: American Families and the Nostalgia Trap.* New York: Basic Books.

Coontz, S. (2005). *Marriage, a History: How Love Conquered Marriage.* New York: Penguin Books.

Coontz, S. (2007). The world historical transformation of marriage. In K. R. Gilbert (Ed.), *The Family: Annual Editions,* (pp. 2-6). Dubuque, Iowa: McGraw-Hill Contemporary Learning Series.

Daedalus (1977). Special issue on the family. 106 (2), *Proceedings of the American Academy of Arts and Sciences.*

Dionne, E.J., Jr. (1991). *Why Americans Hate Politics.* New York: Touchstone Book, Simon & Schuster.

Farganis, S. (1996). *The Social Reconstruction of the Feminine Character* (2nd ed.). Lanham, Maryland: Rowman & Littlefield.

Ferguson, S. J. (Ed.) (2007). *Shifting the Center: Understanding Contemporary Families* (3rd ed.). New York: McGraw-Hill.

Furstenberg, Jr. F. F. (1999/2008). Family change and family diversity. In A. J. Cherlin (Ed.), *Public and Private Families: A Reader* (5th ed.) (pp. 358-370). New York: McGraw-Hill.

Gans, H.J. (1989). Sociology in America: The discipline and the public. American Sociological Association, 1988 Presidential address. *American Sociological Review,* 54 (1), 1-16.

Giddens, A. (1991). *Modernity and Self-Identity.* Stanford, CA: Stanford University Press.

Giddens, A. (1992). *The Transformations of Intimacy.* Stanford, CA: Stanford University Press.

Hutter, M. (1998). *The Changing Family.* Boston: Allyn & Bacon.

Illouz, E. (2007). *Saving the Modern Soul: Therapy, Emotions, and the Culture of Self-Help.* Berkeley, CA: University of California Press.

Jacoby, R. (1987). *The Last Intellectuals: American Culture in the Age of Academe.* New York: Basic Books.

Karpf, F. B. (1932). *American Social Psychology.* New York: McGraw-Hill.

Landis, P. (1958). *Introductory Sociology.* New York: Ronald Press.

Lasch, C. (1977). *Haven in a Heartless World: The Family Besieged.* New York: Basic Books.

Lauer, R.H. & Lauer, J.C. (2007). *Marriage and Family: The Quest for Intimacy* (6th ed.). New York: McGraw-Hill.

Masnick, G. & Bane, M. J. (1980). *The Nation's Families: 1960-1990*. Cambridge, MA: Joint Center for Urban Studies of MIT and Harvard University.

May, E. T. (1999). *Homeward Bound: American Families in the Cold War Era*. New York: Basic Books.

McCarthy, E. D. (1983). Sociology and the changing image of today's family. *Thought*, 58 (228), 93-101.

McCarthy, E. D. (1996). *Knowledge as Culture: The New Sociology of Knowledge*. New York & London: Routledge.

McClay, W. M. (1994). *The Masterless: Self and Society in Modern America*. Chapel Hill & London: The University of North Carolina Press.

Mead, M. (1959). The American family. In H. Smith (Ed.), *The Search for America*. Englewood Cliffs, NJ: Prentice-Hall.

Mills, C.W. (1959). *The Sociological Imagination*. New York: Oxford.

Morgan, S. P. (1996) Characteristic features of American fertility: A description of late twentieth century U.S. fertility trends and differentials. *Population and Development Review* 22, pp. 19-63.

Nisbet, R. (1976). *Sociology as an Art Form*. New York: Oxford University Press.

Oakes, G. (1994). *The Imaginary War: Civil Defense and the American Cold War*. New York: Oxford University Press.

Ogburn, W. F. & Nimkoff, M. F. (1940). *Sociology*. Boston: Houghton Mifflin Co.

Orr, J.B. (1980). The changing family: A social ethical perspective. In V. Tufte & B. Myerhoff (Eds.), *Changing Images of the Family*. New Haven: Yale University Press.

Putnam, R. (2000). *The Collapse and Revival of American Community*. New York: Simon & Schuster.

Riesman, D. with N. Glazer & R. Denney. (1950). *The Lonely Crowd*. New Haven, Connecticut: Yale University Press.

Rose, A.M. (1956). *Sociology: The Study of Human Relations*. New York: Knopf.

Rumney, J. & Maier, J. (1953). *The Science of Society*. New York: Henry Schuman.

Skolnick, A. (1991). *Embattled Paradise: The American Family in an Age of Uncertainty*. New York: Basic Books.

Small, A.W. & Vincent, G. E. (1894). *The Study of Society*. New York: American Book Co.

Spain, D. & Bianchi, S. M. (1996). *Balancing Act: Motherhood, Marriage, and Employment among American Women*. New York: Russell Sage Foundation.

Stacey, J. (1993) Good riddance to "the family": A response to David Popenoe. *Journal of Marriage and the Family* 55 (3), pp. 545-547.

Steiner, G.Y. (1981). *The Futility of Family Policy*. Washington DC: The Brookings Institution.

Uhlenberg, P. (1980). Death and the family. *Journal of Family History*. 5, pp. 313-320.

Veroff, J., Douvan, E., & Kulka, R.A. (1981). *The Inner American: A Self-Portrait from 1957 to 1976*. New York: Basic Books.

Veroff, J., Kulka, R. & Douvan, E. (1981). *Mental Health in America, 1957 to 1976*. New York: Basic Books.

Vidich, A. J. & Bensman, J. (1958). *Small Town in Mass Society*. Princeton, NJ: Princeton University Press.

Wetzel, J. R. (1990). *Monthly Labor Review*, (March), Washington, DC, U.S. Department of Labor, Bureau of Labor Statistics, 4-13.

Williams, R.M. (1951). *American Society*. New York: Knopf.

Wuthnow, R. (1998). *Loose Connections: Civic Involvement in America's Fragmented Communities*. Cambridge, MA: Harvard University Press.

Zaretsky, E. (1986). *Capitalism, the Family, and Personal Life* (revised ed.). New York: Harper & Row.

Zinn, M.B. & Eitzen, D.S. (2005). *Diversity in Families* (7th ed.). Boston: Allyn & Bacon.

5

A Social Constructionist Approach to Therapy with Couples with a Chronic Illness

Joan D. Atwood
Laura Jean Dreher

Abstract

Multiple sclerosis is a chronic, progressive, and degenerative neurological disease which produces a breakdown of the myelin sheath that surrounds central nervous system axons. Recently, there has been an increased recognition of the importance of addressing the counseling needs of MS couples and their families, signaling the need for couple oriented-approaches to address the complex needs of couples coping with MS.

It is the purpose of this chapter to address some of the issues and problems MS couples may experience, taking life cycle issues into consideration. A distinction is made between the illness *experience* and the illness *behavior*. To this we add, the illness *meaning*, the social and psychological definitions given to the illness and the resultant scripts taken on by the couple and by family members. A four-stage therapeutic model based on social constructionist assumptions is then presented and illustrated by case material.

Therapy with Couples with Multiple Sclerosis: A Social Constructionist Approach

The most common acquired neurological disease in the United States and Europe is multiple sclerosis (MS) (Pakenham, 1998). It is a chronic, progressive, and degenerative neurological disease, which produces a demyelization of the axons in the central nervous system, resulting in delayed or blocked neural transmission (Devins & Seland, 1987; Pakenham, 1998). The biopsychosocial model has received significant attention within the last twenty years as a context to address the counseling needs of medical patients and their families. In the past, the counseling needs of couples and families whose members suffer with MS have not received comparable attention as those who endure other chronic illnesses such as cancer, diabetes, and heart disease. Although research is still minimal, there has been an increase in the number of studies regarding the effects of MS symptomology such as fatigue, depression, and cognitive dysfunction on the family (King & Arnett, 2005) and familial interactions with patients diagnosed with MS. Systemically-oriented marital counseling research regarding the needs of MS couples is still lacking, especially in the area of post-modern social constructionist theory. Referral of MS patients, their spouses, and their families to mental health professionals "can be helpful to patients with adjustment difficulties and marital and family dysfunction" (Minden & Moes, 1990, p. 236). Psychotherapeutic interventions including cognitive behavioral and psychopharmacological have been proven to reduce depressive symptoms in MS patients (Mohr, Epstein, Luks, Goodkin, Cox, Goldberg et al, 2003). This treatment modality only addresses the patient and not the family as a system.

The purpose of this chapter is to examine multiple sclerosis and address some of the problems these couples may encounter while considering family life cycle stages (Carter & McGoldrick, 2005). As there has been no research applying social constructionist methods to the condition of MS, this chapter will add the illness *meaning* to the illness *experience* and illness *behavior*. Illness *meaning* is the social and psychological definitions given to the illness and resultant scripts taken on by family members. The illness *experience* is described as the "distress, suffering, and perceived loss of well-being" and the illness *behavior* is defined as "the impaired functioning that is observed by others and is attributed to illness" (Wynne, Shields, & Sirkin, 1992, p.5). Finally, a four-stage therapeutic model based on social constructionist assumptions is presented.

Multiple Sclerosis: The Disease and Related Problems

Etiology of MS is unknown, however, some believe that damage to the central nervous system is a result of attacks by the immune system (Mohr et al, 2003). Lesions on the spinal cord and brain cause patients to experience a variety of physical and/or psychological symptoms. Symptomology varies according to the part of the nervous system that is affected (Ventimiglia, 1986). Diagnosing MS is often a complicated and drawn-out process due to its insidious nature and variety of symptoms. Prognosis is also difficult as the course of this disease is unpredictable.

Patients have been known to live through symptoms that are chronic, progressive and cause rapid deterioration, while most others have experienced symptoms as relapsing and remitting in nature (Bezkor & Canedo, 1987). Approximately 90 percent of MS patients experience a relapsing-remitting course marked by episodic exacerbations that generally partially remit (Warren, Warren, & Cockerill, 1991). Initial onset of symptoms typically occurs in early adulthood. Some studies suggest that symptoms most likely develop between the ages of twenty and forty (McCabe, 2004). These are the ages that people are commonly transitioning through the early stages of the family life cycle (Carter & McGoldrick, 2005) by making decisions about relationships, family planning, and establishing careers; all decisions that will affect their lives (Janssens, de Boer, van Doorn, van der Ploeg, van der Meche, Passchier, & Hintzen, 2003; McCabe, 2004). Besides physical and psychological symptoms, research has also shown that patients suffering from MS are at a higher risk of developing vocational, psychosocial, and interpersonal problems (Long, Glueckauf, & Rasmussen, 1998).

Physical Symptoms

Physical manifestations of the disease include any of the following: debilitating fatigue, vertigo, muscular incoordination (ataxia), paresthesia, numbness and tingling of hands or feet, weakness of one or both legs, loss of vision in one or both eyes (retrobulbar neuritis), double vision (diplopia), impaired speech (dysarthria) with difficulty swallowing, urinary frequency and urgency, loss of bowel and bladder function, frequent bladder and urinary tract infections, and sexual dysfunction (impotence and anorgasmia affect more than 50 percent of men and women) (Sibley, 1990). Fatigue appears to be the most detrimental as it is experienced by 85 percent of MS patients (Skerrett & Moss-Morris, 2006). It impairs instrumental activities of daily living, socialization, and the patient's ability to work. Fatigue is also sometimes related to depression, which is also experienced by MS patients.

Emotional Symptoms

Comorbidity of MS and depression is very common. According to Rao, Huber, and Bornstein (1992), 27 percent to 54 percent of the MS patient population were diagnosed with depressive disorders. "Structural changes in the brain related to demyelination have been suggested as one cause of or contributing factor to depression" (Mohr et al, 2003, p. 1017). MS patients are suggested to have higher rates of depression, suicidality, and low self-esteem as compared to patients with other chronic illnesses (Murray, 1995; Long et al, 1998; Kleiboer, Kuijer, Hox, Jongen, Frequin, & Bensing, 2007). Patients typically present with anger, irritability, worry, and discouragement (Minden & Schiffer, 1990). However, they have also been known to present with anxiety and bipolar disorder. Minden and Schiffer (1990) attribute the manic symptoms related to bipolar disorder to lesions located in the frontal lobes, basal ganglia, and limbic system. The primary assumption related to emotional symptoms and MS is central nervous system damage, however, depression and anxiety might also be related to the uncertainty of the disease's prognosis. "Successful treatment for depression requires that the patient make changes in behavior and thinking patterns" (Mohr et al, 2003, p. 1018).

Cognitive Symptoms

As there are a wide variety of physical and psychological symptoms and an uncertain prognosis associated with MS, patients are often hypervigilant in terms of interpreting bodily sensations. Cognitive distortions of bodily sensations may lead patients to partake in unhelpful behaviors such as overfunctioning or extended inactivity due to fears that they will end up in a wheelchair (Skerrett & Moss-Morris, 2006). Excessive focus on bodily sensations is correlated with increased fatigue and social disability (Skerrett & Moss-Morris, 2006).

Disturbances of recent memory, sustained attention, verbal fluency, conceptual reasoning, and visuospatial perception are most frequently associated with cognitive impairment (Rao, Leo, Bernardin, & Unverzagt, 1991). Loss of cognitive abilities has been shown to impair instrumental activities of daily living and socialization, increase rates of sexual dysfunction, decrease social participation, and decrease the likelihood of employment for MS patients (Rao et al, 1991). According to Mohr et al (2003), a decrease in cognitive functioning may limit the patient's capacity to continue behaviors associated with treatment gains following the cessation of active treatment.

Marital Problems

McCabe (2004) reported that studies have indicated MS strains relationships and couples with MS have less relational satisfaction than those in the general population. King and Arnett (2005) found that depression and fatigue are primary predictors of dyadic maladjustment in MS couples. Depressed and fatigued patients are more likely to pose as a burden on significant others because they are less likely to engage in dynamic marital relationships. Becoming less responsive and more dependent may cause conflict and resentment within the relationship. This study also postulated that problems within the martial relationship increase the amount of fatigue and depression that the patient experiences (King & Arnett, 2005). Pakenham (1998) reported that studies have shown that patients and their caregiver's level of distress significantly correlate, therefore, one might say that the couple responds to illness as a system. Both patient and spouse are affected by the patient's illness, but also by their partner's emotional distress. A reorganization effort is required when illness disrupts the marital/familial system. Kleiboer et al (2007) suggest that due to their depleted psychological resources MS couples are vulnerable to negative interactions. These negative interactions have been correlated with increased end-of-day negative mood for both patient and spouse (Kleiboer et al, 2007). Having dissimilar coping strategies broadens the couple's repertoire and maximizes their ability to respond to the disease (Pakenham, 1998). Prognostic uncertainty leaves the patient in a position of needing to adapt to new circumstances. Not all relationships fail after a partner is diagnosed with MS, some relationships are actually enhanced. King and Arnett (2005) found that better marital adjustment was associated with longer diagnostic duration. This implies that spouses are capable of adapting together to the new demands that the illness presents to the both of them over time.

Sexuality

As aforementioned sexual dysfunction is one of the many physical symptoms experienced by MS patients. Men with MS generally report more occurrence of sexual dysfunction than the general population and also than women with MS, and women with MS report similar levels of sexual problems as women in the general population (McCabe, 2002; McCabe, 2004). Erectile dysfunction is the most commonly-reported sexual symptom for men, which is related to difficulties with masturbation (McCabe, 2002). Although exacerbation of physical symptomology is correlated with increased levels of anxiety and depression, McCabe (2004) did not find an association between exacerbation and sexuality and relationship satisfaction. In fact, she speculates that the exacerbation of symptoms improved relational functioning as the suffering draws partners closer together. Those who do not experience exacerbation are said to have poorer sexual and relational satisfaction (McCabe, 2004). MS is not associated with deterioration in sexuality.

Medication Effects

Currently, there is no cure and symptomatic relief from the disease is minimal (Rao et al, 1992; Pakenham, 1998). Some medications used for the treatment of MS are associated with decreasing libido and/or sexual performance. It is helpful for marriage and family therapists working with MS couples to be aware of the potential side effects related to these medications. Heterocyclic antidepressants have been proven effective in the treatment of both cognitive dysfunction and unipolar depression, but cause additional physical, neurological, and sexual functioning problems for MS patients (Minden & Moes, 1990; Rao et al, 1992; Schiffer & Wineman, 1990), as well as exacerbate cognitive impairment, which could influence the utilization of fantasy during sexuality.

The Social Construction of Illness

Based upon the literature review, much of the writings on multiple sclerosis view the disease through a bio-medical lens meaning that MS is considered an organic disease, caused by a gradual deterioration of the myelin sheath, and currently having no cure. MS is diagnosed using biomedical assessment techniques and the care of the individual is under medical authority, which may involve the prescription of medication and/or hospitalization. However, seeing MS only through a biomedical lens is limiting in that it gives little consideration to the social factors affecting disease definition, experience, and/or progression, including the balance of power in the relationship of caregiver and patient. Using only bio-medical lenses to view the MS can result in the medicalization of the disease, the individual, and the family, which could lead to a justification of control "for the good of the patient." In addition, to using a bio-medical lens, the present authors suggest utilizing a social constructionist approach. For purposes of therapy, it seems that a social constructionist approach is more helpful.

Berger and Luckmann (1966) describe social constructions as the consensual recognition of the coherence or realness of a constructed reality, plus the socialization process by which people acquire this reality. The social constructionist approach believes that all humans participate in social action and interaction, which takes place in a sociocultural environment. This sociocultural environment includes "taken for granted" assumptions, rules, and beliefs about what it means to be sick, to have a disease, etc. It is within this framework of shared definitions that patients and caregivers interact and behave accordingly. And it is this social context that determines individuals' scripts for behavior. Scripts are plans that people have about what they are doing and what they are going to do. They justify situations that are in agreement with them and challenge those that are not. They constitute the available repertoire of socially-recognized acts and statuses, and roles and the rules governing them. Scripts operate at a social, personal, and intrapsychic level (Atwood, 1992). Within this framework, shared knowledge of MS is a collective definition, part of the sociocultural world of the person with MS and that of their caregivers.

MS is a life, which generally requires significant changes in the ongoing life pattern of the individual and his or her family (Holmes and Masuda, 1974). Life events such as MS tend to necessitate a redefinitional process by all family members. This redefinitional process involves the incorporation of the idea that a family member is ill. This is a continual, co-emergent process, which is played out by different family members in different ways. It primarily involves a construction of a reality centered around the concepts of sickness and disease, often involving isolation and control. The "sick" family member becomes more isolated as those who are healthy take on more controlling attributes. The process is painful, not deliberate, yet generally involves the taking in of the symptomatic patient definition.

Therapeutic Considerations

Therapy from a social constructionist position explores the couple's meanings around incidents, behaviors, and encounters with MS and the medical system and how these are determined by the sociocultural environment. It is a therapy of uncertainty in that it assumes that the meanings of behaviors and emotions are relative and suggests that psychological and emotional characteristics are as much a part of the observer's interpretation or assessment as they are characteristics of the persons (Atwood, 1993; 1993a). The therapist is reflective, listens to the couple's language, learns it, and uses it to create a comfortable, "safe" environment. The basic assumption is that the clients are the experts in knowing what is best for them. The role of the therapist is that of curious observer—interested in learning about the couple's story.

1. Joining The Couple's Meaning Systems

The beginning of any therapy involves joining (Minuchin & Fishman, 1974) or the construction of a workable reality (Cimmarusti & Lappin, 1985). This process transforms the definition of the couple's problems from one of a paradigm of individual causality to one of couple interaction. Here the couple sees that the therapist has heard, acknowledged and valued them.

Exploration of Medical History and the Present Symptoms

An integral part of the joining process with an MS couple entails a sensitive exploration of experiences with other professionals who have been involved in diagnosis and treatment. This may provide useful information about prior assessments and attitudes, which may be impacting on the patient and the couple relationship. A thorough discussion with MS couples of previous medical, neurological, and psychological evaluations, as well as prior and current approaches to treatment is critical.

It is important for the therapist to learn the impact of the disease on the couple relationship, including a mutually-informative discussion about the use of all medications and their side effects. In this way the therapist learns how the couple "sees" the MS.

2. Inviting the Couple to Explore Their Meaning Systems

Family of Origin Issues

Issues from one's family of origin may become much more complex in the presence of a chronic illness like MS. According to Bowen (1978), "Chronic illness ... can absorb great quantities of the undifferentiation in a nuclear family and can protect other areas from symptoms" (p.205). A genogram may be useful in tracking the family's meaning systems and scripts around previous illnesses and unanticipated crises and in bringing to light different definitions of illness. Exploration of the different definitions held by the family of origin pertaining to illness and loss in each partner's family of origin may surface. In the context of a chronic illness, the definitions and meanings, which emerge are generally isomorphic to those that existed in both families of origin (Rolland, 1989).

Present Structural Considerations

The complexities of MS often necessitate the use of an integrated approach when exploring an MS couple's counseling needs. Structural issues, such as the permeability of boundaries, the degree of familial closeness, and the role of parental children (Minuchin, 1974) can be considered in the context of both caretaking definitions and demands and available financial resources. Whether it is the principal wage earner who becomes incapacitated or the parent most responsible for child care, support and assistance from family members and close friends may be vitally important. Adaptability and accommodation to the demands of the illness may precipitate or accentuate what the couple defines as enmeshment problems. Rolland (1989) suggests that the occurrence of chronic illness is analogous to the addition of a new member to a family, which sets in motion a centripetal process of socialization to the illness. The ill parent may take on the role of a competing sibling with special needs, losing parental status and creating the semblance of a single-parent family. This situation has the potential to create a parentified child or induct a grandparent into an active parenting role. However the family adjusts its boundaries, it is important to note that the process is a relational dynamic that involves the labeling of the person with MS as the patient.

Self Disclosure

For MS couples, the creation of a therapeutic environment, which emphasizes warmth, empathy, and unconditional positive regard (Rogers, 1961) seems particularly helpful. Loyal, caring, loving, well-meaning behavior can have the potential to become defined as intrusive and over-bearing and in many ways can add to feelings of incompetentcy in the MS patient. Overwhelmed, distressed spouses may find it difficult or feel embarrassed to discuss their own fears, needs, vulnerabilities, or feelings of resentment about the loss of privacy, exclusivity, and intimacy in the relationship. Supporting honest self-disclosure on the part of the non MS spouse may help to rebalance the marital system by empowering the MS spouse to offer comfort and emotional support to his or her partner. An object relations-based approach to couple therapy (Hendrix, 1988; Nichols, 1988; Scharff & Scharff, 1991) may be particularly helpful in this regard, assuming that the level of cognitive functioning is not problematic. In some couples, cognitive distortion processes may increase as a consequence of progressive neurological damage, leaving the well partner even more confused and distressed. In other couples, complicated and sensitive issues of power, control, and dependency may become the focus of couple therapy or the illness may be inducted as a triangulated component of the couple.

Utilizing Imago Relationship Therapy (Hendrix, 1988) and a future oriented relationship vision (Atwood, 1993) may be instrumental in establishing new patterns of communication for the couple, which emphasize mutual validation, empathy, and recognition of their shared sense of loss. Within the context of a "safe" holding environment, it may be possible to address both partners' fears of abandonment and feelings of dependency that may be exaggerated by the disease process. Behavior change requests on the part of the well partner may be novel to the relationship, especially since the onset of the illness. A new balance may be achieved by empowering the patient to reciprocate attention to an unaddressed need of the spouse.

3. Inviting the Couple to Expand Their Meaning Systems

It is not apparent to most individuals that there are alternative ways of behaving. Our meaning systems makes areas outside the dominant ones seem invisible. This invisibility serves to maintain and foster adherence to the dominant definitions. In fact, the function of socialization and of the sanctions against moving outside the dominant script is to keep individuals within it. To find, name, focus on, and help the couple experience alternative meanings and scripts is the intention of this invitation (Atwood, 1993a).

Externalizing the Symptom: What Are the Effects of the Problem?

White's (1989) notion of "exceptions" was originally based in Bateson's idea of restraints—those ideas, events, experiences that are less likely to be noticed by people because they are dissonant with individuals' descriptions of the problem. To meet the challenge of constructing new possibilities with the couple White (1989) suggests "externalizing as an approach to therapy that encourages persons to objectify, and at times, to personify, the problems that they experience as oppressive" (p.5). As the problems become autonomous and external to the individual or the relationship, they may become less fixed and restrictive. The process of relative influence questioning leads to a mapping of the problems' effects "across various interfaces, opening up a very broad field for the search for and identification of unique outcomes" (p.10). A combination of constructionist and cognitive therapeutic techniques may enable couples to make some sense of their tragedy, in part by attributing it to external rather than internal factors (Brooks & Matson, 1982; Ventimiglia, 1986). In addition, some studies indicate that cognitive-behavior therapy is effective in the treatment of depression in MS patients and in the management of distress related to the subjective recognition of lost or diminished intellectual faculties (Halligan, Reznikoff, Friedman, & LaRocca, 1988; Larcombe & Wilson, 1984). In other words, as the couple's view of their realities is explored through the use of questions about exceptions, they ultimately recognize other aspects of their realities where they had experienced success with the problem. In so doing their realities expand.

4. Helping the Couple to Stabilize Their New Meaning Systems

At this point, alternative meaning systems are available to the family and what once was invisible now holds potential for new solutions. The original meaning system, which held the problem has been deconstructed and expanded to include new meanings and new descriptions. The family can now begin to focus on the future. Future focus enables them to visualize their future relationship with the problem. It is helpful for the couple to accept the reality of the problem yet to think of their relationship in terms of "the best it could be." Questions like, "If you could stretch the rubber band three years into the future, what would that look like? How would your family be different? How else would it be different? How would you like it to be?" are helpful.

By asking questions around future trends and choices, the therapist is making that future more real and more stable. As Penn (1985) suggests, when faced with questions about the future— even if that future really only has the status of the hypothetical—"the system is free to create a new map" (p. 300). Questions such as "How will your best future with the problem look?" require speculation about difference and help consolidate the emerging new meaning system for the family. Often rehearsal precedes performance. How will you solve other problems that crop up in the future? Here, a version of de Shazer's (1991) miracle question can be used: "If a miracle were to happen tonight while you were asleep and tomorrow morning you awoke to find that your family could mobilize to solve most problems associated with the MS, what would be different? How would you know that this miracle had taken place? How would each of you be different?"

Another way of stabilizing the new meaning system is put forth by Epston and White (1990) when they discuss how they invite family members to a special meeting where, through questioning, they discuss the person's story of their therapy adventure. The family members are asked to recount how they became aware of their problem and what steps they took to solve it. They can also recount how and which resources they mobilized as they generated solutions to their problems. They can speculate how they will use these resources to solve future problems. Epston and White (1990) believe that here the therapist can ask the family members to recount their transition from perhaps a negativistic one–a view that focused mainly on the problem and loss to one that includes an expanded vision, which includes the problem yet incorporates more mobilizing meanings and definitions. In addition, the therapist also can provide his/her story of the person's therapy adventure and they can then discuss their collaborative efforts, thereby helping to reinforce the notion of a "new meaning system."

Figure 1 outlines the social constructionist approach to therapy discussed in this section.

Case Material

Jen E., 37 and Tom E., 39 have been married for 13 years and have three children: Peter, 10, Susan, 8 and Alana, 3. The couple decided to seek therapy at this time because of Jen's recent MS diagnosis and "the emotional impact it was having on the family."

The couple met in high school and dated throughout college. They married shortly after Jen's graduation. Both Tom and Jen's families of origin welcomed their new in-laws and "comfortable arrangements" were easily made for the sharing of holidays and special occasions: both families expanded to include each other.

Figure 1
Summary of Social Constructionist Therapy with an MS Couple

A SOCIAL CONSTRUCTIONIST APPROACH
TO COUNSELING AN MS COUPLE

JOINING THE COUPLE'S MEANING SYSTEMS

↓

INVITING THE COUPLE TO EXPLORE THEIR
MEANING SYSTEMS

↓

INVITING THE COUPLE TO EXPAND THEIR
MEANING SYSTEMS

↓

HELPING THE COUPLE TO STABILIZE THEIR NEW
MEANING SYSTEMS

Tom is a successful accountant who experiences periods of intense demands on his time, particularly during tax season. Tax time is "normally a very stressful and draining, protracted period of time" for both Tom and Jen, adding additional stresses to Tom who often works sixteen hours a day and Jen who then must cope with familial responsibilities almost single-handedly. Jen is a commercial artist who has worked for the same advertising agency for the past twelve years. Although she has accommodated to the changing needs of her family by working on a part-time basis from her home office, she often has deadlines, which require flexibility in her schedule. Both Jen and Tom's parents live in nearby communities and have been consistently available to help with their grandchildren's activities during these peak times.

Jen experienced her first episode of optic neuritis when she was in her early twenties. She was treated with oral steroids, but developed "serious adverse side effects" and was told by her doctor not to take them again. Subsequently, she went through unexplained periods of exhaustion and bouts of numbness in her leg and arm, as well as recurring optic neuritis. Her fingers would frequently become tingly and numb. During her second pregnancy, she developed a paresthesia in the lower part of her body, which was attributed to "the baby pressing on a nerve." The condition resolved itself after several weeks and no other explanation was sought at that time.

Six months ago Jen had a protracted viral respiratory infection, which left her exhausted and again experiencing numbness in her right leg, arm, and fingers. She was referred for an MRI (Magnetic Resonance Imaging) examination, which revealed evidence of a demyelination process in her brain. The diagnosis of MS was further confirmed by laboratory testing of cerebrospinal fluid following a lumbar puncture. The confirmation of the MS diagnosis was received as "both devastating, terrifying, and a relief to finally know what is wrong—after all this time."

When the couple came in for therapy, they expressed great concern over "the uncertainty of Jen's future and the effect it would have on family life." Tom spoke of his fear of "losing Jen to the MS." Jen was tearful as she voiced her concerns about becoming "disabled, dependent, and a burden" to the people she loved. In the first stage of therapy, the therapist joined with the family's meaning systems. As a curious observer, the therapist listened and learned the family's language and story about the problem and then used this language to join and create a comfortable environment.

The second stage of therapy involved proposing and explaining the notion of a family meaning system and an invitation to the couple to explore their meaning systems. To do this the therapist needed to understand the couple's frame of the problem. Each spouse was asked to tell their story about their own family of origin, with the therapist paying particular attention to their narratives about the incidence of familial illness and their experience of it. Both Jen and Tom discussed their present family relationships and their story about how they "see" their relationship in the future. It was learned through Jen's story that her mother had many opportunities to assume a medical caretaking role, often forsaking her own needs in the service of others. Jen believed that her mother was "the consummate martyr," a role that she did not "wish to emulate." Jen also expressed the belief that her mother was "overprotective" about her health, often encouraging Jen to "stay home and take it easy." She recalled that she often thought it was easier for her mother "to attend to other people's needs than her own." A belief present in Jen's understanding of her mother's focus on other people's health problems related to issues of selfishness versus selflessness. Jen grew up believing that "the children come first, the husband second, and yourself last." It was learned through Jen's story that her mother "always did for others without regard for the toll it took on her." She remembers her mother's "crankiness" and "irritability," which she attributed to the constant fatigue her mother experienced as a consequence of her "chronic over functioning." Jen's story was laden with ambivalence and conflict about the "appropriate role of a wife and mother who has needs of her own." Jen described her father's pride in referring to his wife as "the brick." Jen expressed her concerns that MS would diminish her ability to "fulfill my obligations to my husband and children." Although a successful professional, Jen did not initially address the potential loss of her own artistic abilities or her career, focusing instead on the "price my family will have to pay as a result of my physical limitations." Jen's descriptions of current family life were filled with guilt and self-recrimination for "letting everyone down" and for "feeling like a burden."

Tom's story about life in his family of origin was tinged with sadness and fear. Tom's mother "was sickly" for as long as Tom could remember: "Medically there was always something wrong with Mom. She was in and out of hospitals frequently and at home we had to fend for ourselves and be quiet so she could rest." Tom's mother died of leukemia when he was fourteen. However, Tom's father remarried a year later. He described his stepmother as a "dynamic, warm and vivacious woman whose vitality brought life back into our home and family." Tom was "plagued by memories" of his mother's weakness and dependency and Jen's periods of MS-related exhaustion were "painful reminders." When asked to tell their story about the "emotional impact" on the family, both Jen and Tom agreed that "the unpredictable nature of MS and the uncertainty of its course" leave them feeling "frightened and out of control." Tom felt that since her diagnosis, Jen had withdrawn from him both emotionally and physically.

In the third stage of social constructionist therapy, the couple was invited to expand their meaning systems. This was accomplished by first learning about the Es' story in the present. The goal was to identify what information the couple was selecting from the environment to fit into each of their meaning systems and how it was reinforcing the present system. It was at this time that the couple learned how each one of them inadvertently participated in intensifying and perpetuating "the emotional impact" on the family. When Tom was asked, "How do you think of the problem?," his story was that "history was repeating itself." Tom was consumed with a "sense of inadequacy" and felt "at a loss" as to how he could "make a difference in Jen's life." He recalled the "sense of futility" he felt as his mother's illness progressed. He cried as he remembered his father's "sadness and loneliness" during that time. Tom's strong identification with his father's pain and loss, in conjunction with his own painful memories and losses seemed to be compounding his difficulty in coming to terms with Jen's MS. He described feeling "overwhelmed" at the prospect of caring for Jen and the three children.

Tom also stated that he was "depressed and worried about his ability to deal with the future." When Jen was asked to describe how she thought of the MS in the present, she spoke of the "guilt" she felt for inflicting this "burden" on the family. She cried as she listened to Tom and apologized to him for "reopening old wounds." She described the "inadequacy" she felt as both a wife and mother, particularly when the fatigue left her with "no energy or interest in anything other than resting." She spoke of her mother's "untiring devotion to the family" and said she felt "like a failure for not being able to fulfill the role" her mother had modeled for her. She expressed her belief that her "depression and withdrawal were a function of the impact of the diagnosis." She attributed her "loss of self-esteem" to the "resignation and acceptance" of herself as "the needy sick one." Jen also felt guilty about her "diminished libido," which she believed "deprived Tom of a fully functioning wife." Jen seemed to focus almost entirely on the negative consequences of her illness for the rest of her family, as if the impact on her own life was incidental.

Based on the experiences that Jen and Tom had encountered in their families of origin, each had a different family legacy of familial roles and responsibilities. Prior to Jen's illness, the complementarity of their roles worked well. However, with the intrusion of Jen's illness into their couple relationship, it now became necessary for them to ascribe different meanings to the constructs of wife and mother, and to reconsider their notions of "old family legacies" in the presence of the newly diagnosed MS. The recognition that her mother had modeled martyrdom helped Jen to relinquish some of her unrealistic "Supermom" expectations of herself. The impact of the premature death of Tom's mother had served to activate his fear of abandonment by Jen. It had also generated in him the assumption that serious illness always results in loneliness and a loss of intimacy. He had heightened his awareness of the awesome responsibility that caretaking entails, but his narrative did not reflect any recognition of the self-sufficiency and family bonding that could develop as an outgrowth of their experience.

Assisting the couple to expand their meaning system involved the utilization of exceptions found in their original stories. Tom was asked to recall some happier memories of time his family spent together, including his mother. He smiled as he remembered her "devilish sense of humor," which he believed he "inherited" from her. He also recalled being praised for his ability to "shop, cook, and clean" at a very young age. His mother told him that "with those skills" he would be "any woman's dream come true." Jen laughed and nodded her head in agreement. She told Tom that it gave her "great peace of mind" to know that he could care for their family "so competently." As Tom listened to Jen refer to him as "heroic," he blushed. Clearly, Tom had never considered his adaptive skills to be extraordinary, but Jen did. She spoke of "the strength of Tom's character" and how much she admired Tom's "multifaceted" interests and abilities. Jen then shared her belief that with both Tom and her mother as role models, she constantly felt the need to "prove" herself. As Tom listened, he was "amazed" to hear Jen's characterization of him as "the strong one."

Through the process of externalization of the MS, it was possible to introduce the notion of a powerful and intrusive force that was threatening to interrupt their lives. The strengthening of their couple relationship made it possible for both Jen and Tom to appreciate the power of their combined strengths and fostered a new level of intimacy between them. By mapping the influence of the MS on their lives, it became easier to plan for times when Jen needed to rely on others for help. It also fostered a new camaraderie as the creation of alternative plans came to be viewed as "war games and strategies to beat their enemy: the MS." The familial "sharing" of the MS represented a significant shift in thinking about "Jen's illness." There was no longer an individual dealing with the "emotional impact it was having on the family." Rather, Jen and Tom now thought of themselves as "a couple and a family who were a team and who would grow stronger and closer" because of their shared "problem."

In mapping the influence of MS on the Es' relationship, Jen expressed concerns about her ability to continue to participate fully in her children's activities. She was worried that they would not be able to understand why she could no longer participate in as many of their activities as she once did and believed that as a result they would become angry and resentful of her. She was also concerned about her ability to consistently discipline them. Jen was struggling with many different aspects of her changing role. It is often difficult to recognize and to appreciate normal developmental issues in child rearing when they are viewed within the framework of a serious illness in the family. Raising three young children in a healthy family system can be very demanding and stressful. Helping Jen and Tom to recognize common parenting problems enabled them to "normalize" some of their concerns.

The last stage of therapy was to stabilize the couple's new meaning system. This was accomplished by focusing on the future, a very difficult and uncertain task in the presence of MS. Both Jen and Tom spoke of "new possibilities for closeness" as a result of their more open style of communication. They both expressed their determination to maintain "a mutually supportive" relationship, to "put the MS in its place" when it became too intrusive. Through the use of language, the couple had cocreated a new meaning system. They had empowered themselves to control the design of their own family map.

Summary

There is widespread agreement that marital adjustment is vitally important to the emotional health of individuals with MS. MS can seriously impair marital intimacy, causing both partners great emotional pain. It was the purpose of this chapter to address some of the issues and problems MS couples may experience, taking the biomedical issues into consideration. In so doing, a distinction was made between the illness *experience*, the distress, suffering, and perceived loss of well-being, and illness *behavior*, the impaired functioning that is observed by others and is attributed to illness. The concept of illness *meaning*, the social and psychological definitions given to the illness and the resultant scripts taken on by the family members, was added. A four-stage social constructionist therapeutic model was then presented and illustrated by case material.

References

Atwood, Joan D. (1992). Constructing a sex therapy frame: Ways to help couples deconstruct sexual problems. *Journal of Sex and Marital Therapy*, 18, 3, 196-218.
Atwood, Joan D. and Ruiz, Joan (1993). Social constructionist therapy with the elderly. *Journal of Family Psychotherapy*, 4(1), 1-31.
Atwood, Joan D. (1993a). Social construction couple therapy. *The Family Journal: Counseling and Therapy for Couples and Families*, 1 (2), 116-130.
Berger, P. and Luckman, T. (1966). *The Social Construction of Reality*. New York: Irvington.
Bezkor, M. F., & Canedo, A. (1987). Physiological and psychological factors influencing sexual dysfunction in multiple sclerosis: Parts I & II. *Sexuality and Disability*, 8(3), 143-151.
Bowen, M. (1978). *Family Therapy in Clinical Practice*. Northvale, NJ: Jason Aronson, Inc.
Brooks, N.A., & Matson, R.R. (1982). Social-psychological adjustment to multiple sclerosis: A longitudinal study. *Society of Science and Medicine*, 16, 2129-2135.
Carter, B., & McGoldrick, M. (2005). Overview: The expanded family life cycle. In B. Carter & M. McGoldrick (Eds.), *The Expanded Family Life Cycle: Individual, Family and Social perspectives* (3rd ed., pp. 1 – 26). New York: Allyn & Bacon Classics.
Cimmarusti, R., & Lappin, J. ((1985). Beginning family therapy. *Family Therapy Collections*, 14, 16-25.
De Shazer, S. (1991). *Putting Difference to Work*. New York: Norton.
Devins, G.M., & Seland, T.P. (1987). Emotional impact of multiple sclerosis: Recent findings and suggestions for future research. *Psychological Bulletin*, 101, 363-375.
Epston, D., & White, M. (1990). Consulting your consultants: The documentation of alternative knowledges. *Dulwich Centre Newsletter*, 4.
Halligan, F.R., Reznikoff, M., Friedman, H.P. & LaRocca, N.G. (1988). Cognitive dysfunction and change in multiple sclerosis. *Journal of Clinical Psychology*, 44(4), 540-548.
Hendrix, H. (1988). *Getting the Love You Want*. New York: Harper Perennial.
Holmes, T. H., & Masuda, M. (1974). Life change and illness susceptibility. In B. S. Dohrenwend & B. P. Dohrenwend (Eds.), *Stressful Life Events: Their Nature and Effects* (pp. 45 – 72). New York: John Wiley.
Janssens, A., de Boer, J., van Doorn, P., van der Ploeg, H., van der Meche, F., Passchier, J., & Hintzen, R. (2003). Expectations of wheelchair-dependency in recently diagnosed patients with multiple sclerosis and their partners. *European Journal of Neurology*, 10, 287-293.
King, K. E., & Arnett, P. A. (2005). Predictors of dyadic adjustment in multiple sclerosis. *Multiple Sclerosis*, 11, 700-707.
Kleiboer, A., Kuijer, R., Hox, J., Jongen, P., Frequin, S., & Bensing, J. (2007). Daily negative interactions and mood among patients and partners dealing with multiple sclerosis (MS): The moderating effects of emotional support. *Social Science & Medicine*, 64, 389-400.
Larcombe, N. A., & Wilson, P. H. (1984). An evaluation of cognitive-behavior therapy for depression in patients with multiple sclerosis. *British Journal of Psychiatry*, 145, 366-371.

Long, M. P., Glueckauf, R. L., & Rasmussen, J. L. (1998). Developing family counseling interventions for adults with episodic neurological disabilities: Presenting
problems, persons involved, and problem severity. *Rehabilitation Psychology*, 43(2),
101-117.

McCabe, M. P. (2002). Relationship functioning and sexuality among people with multiple
sclerosis. *Journal of Sex Research*, 39 (9), 302-309.

McCabe, M. P. (2004). Exacerbation of symptoms among people with multiple sclerosis:
Impact on sexuality and relationship over time. *Archives of Sexual Behavior*, 33(6),
593 - 601.

Minden, S.L., & Moes, E. (1990). A psychiatric perspective. In S.M. Rao (Ed.),
Neurobehavioral Aspects of Multiple Sclerosis (pp. 230-250). New York: Oxford
University Press.

Minden, S. L., & Schiffer, R. B. (1990). Affective disorders in multiple sclerosis: Review
and recommendations for clinical research. *Archives of Neurology*, 47, 98-10.

Minuchin, S. (1974). Families and family therapy. Cambridge: Harvard.

Minuchin, S. & Fishman, C. (1974). *Family Therapy Techniques.*Cambridge: Harvard
University Press.

Mohr, D. C., Epstein, L., Luks, T. L., Goodkin, D., Cox, D., Goldberg, A., Chin, C.,
& Nelson, S. (2003). Brain lesion volume and neuropsychological function predict
efficacy of treatment for depression in multiple sclerosis. *Journal of Consulting and
Clinical Psychology*, 71 (6), 1017-1024.

Murray, T. J. (1995). The psychosocial aspects of multiple sclerosis. *Neurology Clinics*,
13(1), 197-223.

Nichols, W.C. (1988). *Marital Therapy.* New York: Guilford Press.

Pakenham, K. (1998). Couple coping and adjustment to multiple sclerosis in care re-
ceiver-carer dyads. *Family Relations*, 47 (3), 269-277.

Rao, S. M., Huber, S. J., & Bornstein, R. A. (1992). Emotional changes with multiple
sclerosis and Parkinson's disease. *Journal of Consulting and Clinical Psychology*,
60 (3), 369-378.

Rao, S. M., Leo, G. J., Bernardin, L., & Unverzagt, F. (1991). Cognitive dysfunction in
multiple sclerosis: 1. Frequency, patterns, and predictions. *Neurology*, 41, 685-691.

Rogers, C.R. (1961). *On Becoming a Person: A Therapist's View of Psychotherapy.*
Boston: Houghton Mifflin.

Rolland, J.R. (1989). Chronic illness and the family life cycle. In B. Carter & M.
McGoldrick, (Eds.), *The Changing Family Life Cycle*, pp. 433-456. Boston: Allyn
and Bacon.

Scharff, D. E. & Scharff, J. S. (1991). *Object Relations Couple Therapy.* Northvale, NJ:
Jason Aronson, Inc.

Schiffer, R. B., & Wineman, N. M. (1990). Antidepressant pharmaco-therapy of
depression associated with multiple sclerosis. *American Journal of Psychiatry*, 147,
1493-1497.

Sibley, W. A. (1990). Diagnosis and course of multiple sclerosis. In S. M. Rao (Ed.),
Neurobehavioral Aspects of Multiple Sclerosis (pp. 5-14). New York: Oxford
University Press.

Skerrett, T. N., & Moss-Morris, R. (2006). Fatigue and social impairment in multiple
sclerosis: The role of patients' cognitive and behavioral responses to their symptoms.
Journal of Psychosomatic Research, 61, 587-593.

Ventimiglia, J. (1986). Helping couples with neurological disabilities: a job description
for clinical sociologists. *Clinical Sociology Review*, 4, 123-139.

Warren, S., Warren, K. G., & Cockerill, R. (1991). Emotional stress and coping in multiple
sclerosis (ms) exacerbations. *Journal of Psychosomatic Research*, 35(1), 37-47.

White, M. (1989). The externalizing of the problem and the reauthoring of lives and relationships. *Selected Papers*. Adelaide: Dulwich Centre Publications.

Wynne, Shields, & Sirkin (1992). Illness, family theory, and family therapy: 1. Conceptual issues. *Family Process*, 3-18.

6

Chronic Illness: An Inquiry into Understanding Irritable Bowel Syndrome from a Place of Uncertainty

Mary E. Canzoneri

Abstract

This chapter discusses the definition of Irritable Bowel Syndrome (IBS), its impact on individuals, couples, and families taking into consideration cultural factors, economic factors, life cycle issues, and traditional medical models. Deficit assumptions surrounding therapy with the chronically ill, including the psyshosomatic model, standardized family assessments, family of origin issues, object relations and solution-focused models of therapy are explored. Social constructionism as it relates to narrative therapy is presented as a both/and world view within which to effectively create possibilities for IBS sufferers.

Irritable Bowel Syndrome

Irritable Bowel Syndrome (IBS) is considered a functional gastrointestinal (GI) disorder, a common and troublesome condition. IBS is a chronic or recurrent disorder not explained by structural or biochemical abnormalities (Salt, 1995, 2002). Approximately 35 million people are affected in the United States, one out of five people are affected by this disorder including children, young adults, the middle-aged, and the elderly. The average age of onset is 20-29 years of age (Salt, 1995, 2002; Burstall, et al, 1998). Symptoms of IBS include chest pain, indigestion, nausea, vomiting, pain in the pelvis area, diarrhea, constipation, and bowel incontinence.

The symptoms of IBS can be triggered by a number of things, such as, foods; caffeine; stress; seasonal changes; hormones; psychological problems; or drugs and medication. These symptoms appear to come and go over time—often triggered or worsened by dietary factors and stress (Burstall, 1998; Salt and Nemark, 1995, 2002). Psychological stress or emotional responses to life stress can influence GI function in anyone and can produce GI symptoms such as pain or altered bowel function. Psychological problems are not the cause of functional disorders but rather serve to exacerbate the symptoms (Salt, 1995). Many people with IBS also suffer from what has been called "irritable body" or what doctors call somatization. Bodily symptoms often associated with IBS include but are not limited to: fatigue and low energy; insomnia; headaches; dizziness; decreased sex drive; difficulty concentrating; and shortness of breath.

IBS creates psychological consequences such as a reduced sense of health and well-being; a constant concern about symptoms and how to control them; problems with daily living; problems with interpersonal relationships; and disability resulting in missed work days—IBS is the second leading cause of industrial absenteeism in the United States (Lorenz, 1994). There can also exist a vicious circle of stress, symptoms, and psychology because of the lack of control over bowel movements experienced by IBS sufferers. An individual may worry constantly over his or her IBS and because of the worrying, the body reacts with stress symptoms and this can trigger the IBS symptoms (Salt, 1995, Salt and Neimark, 2002).

IBS is not diagnosable by any medical means and therefore difficult to treat with anything other than over-the-counter medicines (Burstall, et al, 1998; Salt, 1995, Salt and Neimark, 2002). The individual's self-esteem may gradually show signs of erosion and negative self-perception following embarrassing chronic illness encounters (Livneh & Antonak 2005). In order to avoid stress, some individuals with IBS may withdraw from many social activities (Falvo, 1991). Sufferers of this disorder may be embarrassed because of the nature of the disorder and because of the uncertainty of symptoms may choose to remain socially isolated.

Demands of Chronic Illness

Individual

As an individual, a chronically-ill person has a myriad of issues to deal with on a daily basis. One of the first questions of the "newly un-healthy" ask is, "Why me?" This poses a dilemma because you may feel as if you have been given only two choices for the answer: (1) you are special and have been chosen to transcend ordinary human experience or (2) you are deficient and have been given the deficiency to atone for your deficiency (Register, 1987, 1999). These are not actually choices but rather are "life limiting" views that have the potential to consume the person into only an "illness." This anxiety of being consumed is a daily event that accompanies any chronic illness. Chronic illness and disability produce significant changes and consequences because individuals must deal with a change of customary lifestyle, loss of control, disruption of a physiological process, pain or discomfort, and potential loss of role, status, independence and financial stability (Falvo, 2005). IBS is already factoring in a certain amount of anxiety and to deal with identity fluctuations will only increase the symptoms, and so another vicious cycle occurs. The concern is that you will be determined by what is wrong with you rather than who you are (Register, 1987, 1999).

If a person becomes subsumed by his or her chronic illness than he or she loses his or her ability to maintain a "self" in the face of an illness. This also relates to a person's ability to deal effectively with his or her chronic illness and maintain power over it. There is a need to understand how people are made subjects or are placed in a particular position that constrains or restricts their actions. Suffering from a chronic illness is easily a restricting event and an individual may feel a loss of power because of the illness. "Power over" is the ability of one person (in this case, illness) to exert control over another and "power to" is the empowerment of personal authority. For a sufferer of IBS, power over becomes a daily battle because of many social issues around controlling bowel functions. This emphasis of power over began in toddlerhood and for IBS sufferers they have lost their power over one of the first bodily functions they learned to control. IBS now has power over them. Power over, however, is inconsistent with relational equality (Rampage, 1994) and if a person wishes to maintain an identity of *who* he or she is rather than *what* he or she is, power becomes a factor in maintaining/regaining his or her "self."

Couple

To understand fully power relations around chronic illness, it is necessary to explore the effect of the wider context of the individual, i.e., spouse or other family members (Towns, 1994). Because the couple relationship is a sexual one, IBS will affect it differently than any other family relationship (Revenson, 1994). Every aspect of a couple's relationship can be affected by a chronic illness on daily basis, from shopping for groceries to sex. A partner who suffers from IBS may have to monitor how long he or she is away from a bathroom, what exactly to eat or not to eat, or may be concerned about loss of bowel control during sex. These feelings and fears can be very limiting to the relationship. The partner may feel shame or guilt about how the illness limits their life together and also limits the other partner's life (Register, 1987, 1999). This can be a most troubling feature to a relationship because the "ill partner" may feel that he or she brings less to the marital relationship than the healthy partner does (Donoghue & Siegel, 1992; Register, 1987, 1999; & Revenson, 1994). There must be a great shame and guilt in believing that you are depriving your spouse of a chance for basic human fulfillment.

It is not certain that a relationship will be affected in any particular way. It is difficult to determine just how a couple relationship will be affected because the relationship itself is a precarious institution, given to constant buffeting by many forces (Register, 1987, 1999). Additionally, there is evidence that physical illness may decrease or increase or be unrelated to marital satisfaction (Schmaling & Sher, 2000). However, certain needs are basic in a relationship and if those needs are not being met, the relationship may be strained. Just as mutual needs being met creates a solid base of satisfaction between people, needs not met on both sides tear away at the fabric of a relationship (Donoghue & Seigel, 1992). Support for a partner with IBS is essential for a relationship to be satisfying. But this may difficult for a spouse whose partner is constantly ill, his or her ability to be an effective support may be constrained because of the constant pressure to do so (Revenson, 1994). He or she may simply get worn down.

A couple's experience of chronic illness also depends on the gender of the "ill partner." Illness can highlight and compound the differences that gender makes. Whether they are the patient or the caregiver, women assume a disproportionate share of the responsibility for maintaining the relationship and providing nurturance (Revenson, 1994). The expectations for men and women are different and so the responses to an illness are different. Women tend to be socialized into caretaking roles in close relationships and are more responsive to the well-being of others (Gilligan, 1982) and tend to experience more burden and psychological stress in the caregiving role (Marks, et al, 2002). It has also been demonstrated that spousal caregivers have been found to experience more negative effects from caregiving than other caregiving relationships (Biegel et al, 1991; George & Gwyther, 1986; Seltzer & Li, 2000; Young & Kahana, 1989). And so the story of an illness will have both his and her versions.

Family

The family influence of a person suffering from a chronic illness is an important element in determining how the individual will cope with his or her illness, whether or not he or she will follow a medical regime, and what, if any, role changes will take place. Wishful thinking, unrealistic expectations of full or immediate recovery and at times blatant neglect of medical advice and therapeutic and rehabilitation recommendation are all examples of noncompliance (Livneh & Antonak, 2005). Noncompliance with medical regimes has been linked to significant others as they act as models and normative influences as well as having the potential to exert more direct control over lifestyle factors (Burg & Seeman, 1994). Stress of chronic illness can derail functioning of a family system with ripple effects to all members and their relationships (Walsh, 2003). These ties can serve as a source of conflict, envy, frustration, devaluation, and demand—all negative and anxiety-provoking influences for a person suffering from IBS.

A family's response to illness can vary from extreme denial to extreme submersion into the illness. The response to an illness depends on the family's configuration and coping skills available as a family system (Donoghue & Seigel, 1992; Register, 1987; & Rolland, 1989; Walsh, 2003). With IBS and other chronic illnesses, some of the coping that is required involves changing roles. If the person who originally drove a family member on a five-hour trip each month now suffers from IBS, this trip may no longer be possible for him or her. This is a concrete example of a role change, other changes are not so obvious. The less obvious role changes involve a person's sense of self and to change this type of role can be threatening to this sense of self (Donoghue & Siegel, 1992). An example of this is the gender-based roles that cast a woman as a caretaker. If the caretaker becomes ill, she must then learn to allow others to care for her as well as know her limits with regard to her illness. A difficult task because of social pressure for a woman to maintain the emotional stability of the family and care for it's members, at all costs to her own sense of self (Gilligan, 1982). Her sense of individual and familial self is being threatened because of IBS and her inability to perform her "role."

As the role changes take place within the person suffering from IBS, whether male or female, other shifts around him or her will also take place. When one family member changes roles, it puts pressure on the others in the family to change (Donoghue & Seigel, 1992, Walsh, 2003).

This creates a system shifting, which may or may not be able to handle such structural changes. Structural realignment will be discussed in further detail in a later section.

In addition to roles affecting how a family will react, the possibility of reactivating painful memories of loss (Walsh., 2003), family legacies of loss and illness as well as belief systems will also shape the coping response (Rolland, 1994; Walsh, 2003). If a family's response around chronic illness is to hold fast to the "pre-illness" structure, there will be no room for change and the family's coping will be in a state of denial. Also important to consider are the expected psychosocial demands of an illness over time in relation to family system dynamics (Rolland, 1989; Rolland & Williams, 2005). The family's response has many facets and many variables to consider when determining in which direction the family will move. All of these considerations are based on belief systems that are in place and are socially constructed and, perhaps unbeknownst to the family, their decision will be made for them if an active role is not taken.

Chronic Illness Etiquette

Sociological Considerations

From a sociological perspective, a person with a chronic illness may be dealing with a "dual prescription." He or she is expected to be psychologically capable of both periods of illness and periods of relative health—society expects flexibility (Register, 1987). In a sense, the person's behavior is supposed to remain in sync with what society deems is the role and this role will fluctuate depending on the health status of the individual. While illness can bring secondary rewards or gains, often if the person does not appear ill, as can be the case with IBS, these benefits are not offered because he or she is not operating within the sick role behavior (Rice, 1992). Human beings operate within a social context and this context can either be a source of stress or comfort in the face of changes (Burg & Seeman, 1994). Clearly, societal demands of constant role changing are too difficult and an IBS sufferer must find a way to incorporate his or her own sense of self as the main focus rather than the illness.

Dealing with chronic illness has numerous daily obstacles including basic conversational habits. Prior to an illness these habits were probably not given extra thought, now they can become a constant source of stress and silent deliberation. While exchanging normal greetings with a person, it is serious breach of etiquette to expose the realities of chronic illness to someone who simply asked the standard "how are you" greeting (Register, 1987). Another source of discomfort is trying to determine if the "asker" actually wants the truth or if he or she just being polite. In addition to this concern, constant attention can cause discomfort. This constant attention can make the person's health loom larger in his or her consciousness and lend a disproportionate significance to his or her life (Register, 1987).

Cultural Norms

In determining how a person may react to his or her chronic illness, it is necessary to learn a considerable amount about his or her culture. Consideration of attitudes, perceptions and behavior within a cultural context is imperative to understanding the chronic illness etiquette. All persons are cultural beings and all attitudes, perceptions, and behaviors gain their meaning from culture (Hardy, 1993). The meaning of adversity and beliefs about what can be done vary with different cultural norms; some are fatalistic while others stress personal responsibility and agency (Walsh, 1998). Western culture is governed and regulated by economics. In a society where employers/ jobs have become the priority in family life, it is not surprising that hiring a person with a chronic illness is considered a "bad decision." From the employer's standpoint, hiring a person whose health is in question is economic carelessness (Register, 1987). For the chronically ill, the force of the work ethic is compounded by the stigma associated with being different (Revenson, 1994). This is a socially constructed dual prescription involving, in this case, the employer and the employee.

Remaining employed can be a positive albeit necessary experience for a person suffering from IBS. Because western culture is steeped in the world of career and money, feelings of self-worth and importance can derive from being employed. Practically, persistent unemployment or loss of the breadwinner can be devastating, a serious chronic illness can drain a family's economic resources (Walsh, 2003). Apart from an economic necessity and the authority of cultural norms, there are sound motives to keep working, even at a much reduced capacity (Towns, 1994; Wilday & Dovey, 2005). Work is after all, the human enterprise. A job can provide structure for a person's life, a sense of satisfaction and productivity from completing meaningful tasks, a feeling of belonging to a valued reference group, a basis of self-esteem and personal identity, and a way to earn one's economic place in society (Moos, 1988). The routine of work and its tangible products provide a safety valve for the anxiety that illness arouses (Register, 1987, 1999). If a person is unable to do these things, either fir him—or herself—or in pursuit of goals, then the sense of well-being is under attack and the individual is likely to be unhappy – happiness is an important part of a healthy lifestyle (Christiansen, 2001). The knowledge that he or she is performing a job up to standard is comforting, because his or her body is no longer performing up to this level. This comfort may alleviate some of the embarrassment experienced with IBS.

Life Cycle Considerations

A chronic illness has a life cycle of its own similar to that of adolescence. When IBS is initially diagnosed, there is a "crisis phase" in which the family will find itself. The family needs to create meaning around the illness that maximizes a preservation of a sense of mastery and competency (Rolland, 1989). The family also grieves for its pre-illness identity while attempting to move toward a position of acceptance of permanent change (Rolland, 1994). It is necessary to reevaluate previous patterns of relating and develop new ones that fit the current situation of a chronic illness, i.e., role changes (Rolland, 1989; Walsh, 2003). Within the context of significant adversity this involves fostering positive role adaptations (Luthar, et al, 2000 and Walsh, 2003). These new patterns should fit the new illness-related developmental demands and also be maintained with a degree of uncertainty and flexibility.

In addition to the state of uncertainty and flexibility, the individual must incorporate developmental tasks of living with a chronic illness and living out other parts of his or her life. These tasks must be brought together into one coherent life structure while still maintaining a sense of self (Rolland, 1989). The transition into the chronic phase of IBS must emphasize autonomy and the creation of a viable ongoing life structure adapted to the realities of the illness (Rolland, 1994). The family must adapt to the realities of chronic illness and create family structures, which accommodate to these realities.

Traditional Medical Models

The biological/medical model assumes that there are distinct differences between the mind and the body. The medical system concerns itself with the biological treatment of an illness and little clinical attention is paid to the person's mental health and his or her family (Rolland, 1994). Recently there has been growing interest in advocating for health care that attends to physical and psychosocial challenges of major health conditions for all family members (Rolland & Walsh, 2005). However, the medical model is still a long way from making the family a priority in the treatment of chronic illnesses.

IBS is not a medically diagnosable disorder, there are no blood tests or X-rays that will prove its existence. This leaves the sufferer of the disorder in another world of uncertainty. There are no prescriptions that are specifically for this disorder and many feel it is purely a psychological illness (Salt, 1995). Years ago people thought IBS was a psychological disorder, but it was not very well-understood (Brandt, 2003). The mind-body connection is emphasized with IBS. Persons with this disorder are taught about the triggers of their illness and ways to avoid the symptoms, as discussed earlier. It is suggested that stress and fatigue have some direct effect on the digestive system (Falvo, 1991; Salt & Neimark, 2002). Psychological factors may aggravate this illness and individuals with this illness compound their stress because they may fear embarrassment and social ridicule as result of their problems with elimination (Falvo, 1991, Wilkinson, 2003).

One of the ways to avoid the symptoms of this illness is by monitoring food intake very carefully. Unfortunately, this may cause a sense of discomfort in social settings because eating is often associated with pleasure and social interaction (Falvo, 1991). An IBS sufferer deals with issues of social stigma and because of the nature of his or her illness cannot enjoy social gatherings to the extent that others can, and may also have difficulty in the workplace because of frequent absences. Research into the sick role behavior shows that the degree to which illness is understood by society and consequences of societal norms for its management play an essential role in the coping response to an illness (Wilday & Dovey, 2005). To compound these issues is the uncertainty under which an individual lives due to the lack of medical answers for the illness. Seeing a chronic illness through only a biomedical lens is limiting in that it gives little consideration to social affects of the disease definition, experience, and/or progression, including the balance of power in the relationship between caregiver and patient (Atwood, 1997; Rolland, 1994).

Deficits of Traditional Approaches

The Psychosomatic Model

The psychosomatic model of understanding families with a chronic illness is based on Minuchin's typology for the family. The illness exists because of system malfunctioning and is maintained through the reciprocal relationships that enable the illness. The psychosomatic family is characterized by excessive over involvement of family members with each other and rigidity in making change when circumstances are warranted (Minuchin, 1975). Because families have a powerful influence on health, equal to traditional medical risk factors (Campbell, 2003), family may or may not be a support during the periods of illness, but this model approaches from the angle that the family system works together to maintain and sometimes create an illness. Although family is most frequently viewed as offering support, there is considerable reason to propose that the family may unwittingly promote the symptomatic expression of the disease (Kerns & Weiss, 1994).

In this model, the family promotes the symptoms of the disease and possibly participates in the onset of the illness itself. When viewing a family through the lens of this model, it is difficult to disentangle which characteristics of individuals or family preexisted the chronic illness diagnosis and which emerged in response to the presence of the chronic condition (Campbell, 2003; Patterson & Garwick, 1994). It is thought that the development of the sick role is in response to societal or at least significant others' expectations of the individual (Kerns & Weiss, 1994). This model focuses only on what is seen through the structural/systemic lens and the views of the family members are not considered when making a hypothesis about the family system.

Assessment of Family Functioning

Olson (1979) developed an early model of assessment specific to families that emphasizes cohesion among family members in its various forms and states. Cohesion can be defined as the emotional bonding family members have with one another and the degree of individual autonomy a person experiences in the family system (Beavers & Voeller, 1983). Autonomy is the other variable that is measured when determining the functionality of family. Based on the Circumplex model, high levels of cohesion (enmeshed) and low levels of cohesion (disengaged) can be problematic (Olson, Russell, & Sprenkle, 1989). Olson, Portner, and Lavee (1985) developed the FACES III instrument composed of two scales—cohesion and adaptability—that operationalize the circumplex model dimensions (Ben-David & Jurich, 1993). From the "expert" stance, a family that can maintain balance and not fall into the extreme categories will be the most adaptable.

According to Olson, Russell, & Sprenkle (1989), higher levels of cohesion and change seem to be associated with higher functioning.

A family with this combination of skills facing a chronic illness would be the most successful at negotiating communication among its' family members and with external systems. If a family communicates clearly within the system, no mixed messages, acts and responds with kindness and support to name a few examples, they will restructure themselves as needed and reach out to external sources.

There have been many attempts to determine a family's response to a stressful event. The Double ABCX model introduced by Hill (1958) and further expanded into the Family Stress and Adaptation Theory (Boss, 2001; McCubbin, McCubbin, & Thompson, 1995; McCubbin & Patterson, 1983; Patterson, 1988) has been widely accepted as a means to assess a family's level of functioning given a crisis. Rather than focusing on the stress event itself, the model(s) focuses on the family's response to the event while considering multiple variables through which the family is responding. Taking into account the build up of stress that may exist, whether or not the family has resources available to deal with stress, how the family perceives stress and what history of stressful events exists together will determine the outcome of the family's adaptation (McCubbin et al, 1980). In this model, four central constructs are emphasized: families engage in active processes to balance family demands with family capabilities as these interact with family meanings to arrive at a family adjustment or adaptation (Patterson, 1988).

When faced with a chronic illness a family may have difficulty shifting power structures, role relationships and relationship rules in response to this stress (Beavers & Voeller, 1983). These two dimensions are placed on a continuum and the therapist determines where on the continuum the family will be placed. Both are seen as important to the family if the family operates within the optimal central area of the continuum, pathology arises in those families operating at either extreme (Beavers & Voeller, 1983). The therapist will determine where on the spectrum the family lies thereby deciding the functioning level of the family.

Beavers (1983) has also developed a model based on a family's "dysfunction." This model places families into various categories depending on their levels of intimacy, power struggles, adaptability, and control issues. There is an "optimal family," an "adequate family," and a "mid range family." The structure, flexibility, and competence of a family are scored and placed within a particular family style (Beavers & Voeller, 1983, Hampson, Hulgus & Beavers, 1991). The ability to change is the criterion for being placed into either an "optimal" family or only a "mid range" family. When a family is not bound to rigid behavior, patterns and responses, it has more freedom to evolve and differentiate (Beavers & Voeller, 1983) and its flexibility is a core process in resilience (Walsh, 2003).

In traditional types of therapy, such as the psychosomatic model, it is thought that assessment of the family/client was the sole job of the "expert" therapist. While the author recognizes the self-report subscales within these assessments, there still exists the overarching view of therapist as "expert." This may follow suit with how IBS sufferers are treated elsewhere, medial settings, places of employment, etc. Because a person is viewed as "deficient" if he or she is ill, the normal societal reaction is to seek "professional" help so the professional can determine what is "wrong." A person with IBS is constantly being assessed, judged, considered, or studied by all of those involved including family members, loved ones, and friends.

The categories developed by standardized assessments, while helpful for research purposes, allow for simplification of the evaluation process for the therapist, may also create a single lens through which the clinician views a family. Using the results of standardized theoretically- and empirically-based methods of assessment to determine and implement specific interventions is difficult but ongoing (Beavers & Hampson, 1990; Olson, Russell, & Sprenkle, 1989; Snyder et al, 1995). They may also serve to perpetuate the cycle of limiting behaviors, which occurs in society at large as well as in the medical and mental health communities. Each family must be respected as a "unique system and assessed and treated with regard to its unique conditions and relationships" (Olson, 1995). To place the families within a category that defines their behaviors and feelings, past, present, and future, defines their reality for them and offers no room for chance, change, or possibility.

Loss of Self within the System

For the chronically ill, loss of self within the medical system, the family system, the couple system, the societal system, or the disease system is a core issue. To no longer feel power or a sense of self is a frightening experience and IBS sufferers may experience this on a daily basis. If the individual is able to retain a certain amount of control than he or she will be more able and willing to accept offers of help from others without feeling diminished by the dependence (Register, 1987, 1999). That sense of control is more than a mere mood or attitude and may well be a vital pathway between the brain, endocrine system, and immune system (Salt & Neimark, 2002). Others may experience help from others as a threat to their sense of independence and competence. He or she may feel that his or her partner is regulating an aspect of his or her life that could be under the control of the owner of this aspect (Revenson, 1994). There may be a feeling of being controlled or monitored and this might be interpreted as others viewing him or her as deficient and incapable.

Families also experience the feelings of being incapable or incompetent because of the treatment they may receive. Relationships with medical staff, insurance staff, and other professionals may lead to these feelings because generally the family's opinions are not considered. These relationships also have unclear boundaries and this can increase the risk of conflict and dissolution in the family system further exacerbating the problem (Rolland, 1994; Patterson & Garwick, 1994). Unfortunatetly there seems to be a failure to communicate and a lack of open dialogue and this widening gap may lead to frustrations with the impersonality of care (Salt & Neimark, 2002). The family may feel overdirected by professionals and underutilized for information about the family system.

Structural Realignment

The nature of chronic illness lends itself to a great deal of change for an individual and a couple/family system. Role changes must occur, flexibility must be a part of the system, and system autonomy must be maintained. However, chronic illness creates a role ambiguity within a system because the loss is ambiguous (Patterson & Garwick, 1994). It is difficult to determine what exactly has been lost when the illness itself remains somewhat of a mystery. This is particularly true with IBS because of the uncertainty of its diagnosis.

Role changes taking place will also do so with a certain amount of ambiguity because of the unknowing nature of future roles. These scripts have not yet been written and it is difficult to know a role without first reading the script. These changes in role responsibilities may very well be outside of traditional gender roles (Revenson, 1994). A couple system will have to work with uncertainty both in the illness and also in the illness roles.

Permeability of a family system is also an important factor in determining the functioning of a system. The family must have a degree of permeability in order to take in the new roles associated with the illness as well as the multitude of relationships that become a daily part of family life (Patterson & Garwick, 1994). Many families facing chronic illness tend to be dominated by the illness and it may take over the family's identity (Campbell, 2003). This realignment will occur because of the introduction of the illness, the medical professionals, and others. The permeability allows the other systems into the family system and the family system autonomy allows the family to maintain its sense of self on a broader level while assisting members in maintaining their individual sense of self.

Family of Origin

For the individual with IBS and his or her partner, family of origin issues can be of significant relevance to capabilities around dealing with a chronic illness. By collecting information about each adult's family of origin, one can anticipate potential areas of conflict and competencies (Rolland, 1989). Early life events can alter the responsiveness of the mind body spirit connection to stress and may lead an individual to being more susceptible to bad stress responses (Salt & Neimark, 2002). Roles that were played out in childhood can become active again if the situation triggers a particular response in one or both partners. It is believed that any psychic energy that is within a person will find a way out through some type of triggering event. This energy is like steam in a boiler, it can only be diverted or discharged (Hamilton, 1989). So, the energy from early childhood interactions may be diverted only to then resurface when needs are not being met later in life.

Drives, which have been said to determine a child's wants and needs, may have been frustrated in early childhood and will now lead to peculiarities of civilized behavior as well as pathological behavior (Hamilton, 1989). For IBS sufferers, gut feelings are based on previous life experience that is also associated with gut sensations—it has been proposed that part or most of our rational decision making may be based upon the imprinted emotional content of prior experiences (Damasio, 1994). Whether these unmet needs are the needs of the "ill" partner or not, in either case this can lead to further disruption of the couple system in addition to the problems associated with IBS.

Overview

The preceding models/theories concerning chronic illness and systems are to be respected in their own right, however, they are deficit views of a family/couple system. These models focus on what is wrong with the client, what is the best diagnosis/category to fit him or her into, and what the expert therapist can do to "fix" the "broken" person or system.

Deficits of Solution-Focused Assumptions

Solution-focused models of viewing client systems mobilize the strengths of the system or individual and focuses solely on those strengths and resources. Any system that is in therapy has coalesced around some "problem" (Anderson & Goolishian, 1992) and this problem is normally the focus of the therapeutic endeavor. A solution-focused orientation is concerned with coalescing around solutions that are already present but may not be noticed. Where the therapist put his or her attention and directs inquiries will inevitably influence the course of treatment and the data that emerge (O'Hanlon, 1992). If the therapist then directs attention to solutions and competencies, these will become the arena in which client and therapist collaborate.

Focusing on what is wrong with people can have a discouraging effect and people will tend to see themselves as sick and damaged, they often forget the resources, strengths, and capabilities they have (O'Hanlon, 1992). Solution-focused models focus on a client's strengths and resiliencies, examining previous solution and exceptions to the problem and then through a series of interventions, encouraging clients to do more of those behaviors (Trepper, et al, 2006). In this view the therapist attempts to change the lens through which the client is looking at his or her life circumstances. The therapist' job is to create a context in which clients gain access to their resources and competence (deShazer, 1991; O'Hanlon, 1992). The lens becomes one of strength and resources already present but unable to be viewed by the client.

The therapist is introducing preexisting ideas to the client but reframing them in ways so as to accentuate the positive contribution he or she made to the event. The process of solution development can be summed up as helping an unrecognized difference become a difference that makes a difference (deShazer, 1991). These exceptions existed and the therapy represents a training to begin to notice these exceptions. On a broader level, exceptions are unique outcomes when they include both the client's feelings and behaviors (Nicholson, 1995). Exploring in more detail the exceptions creates a reality/truth base to these notions and lays a foundation upon which a client places his or her newly-erected lens.

The therapist does not attempt to understand the problems of the client since that would be a "problem-focused" avenue. The therapist moves in a direction away from trying to understand the client's problem and tries to design a solution to it. Designing a solution to this involves questioning the client about their own goals and about exploring themselves as potential resources for problem-solving (Atwood, 1996). The solution exists within the client, waiting to be discovered through a series of solution-oriented questions.

In exploring solutions with the client, the presenting problem is not an area that becomes involved. The therapist does not address this issue with the client, but rather moves into focusing solutions. This may leave the client feeling unvalidated and unheard. In dealing with an IBS sufferer this can further lower feelings of self-worth. In the therapist's enthusiasm to identify exceptions and facilitate change, he or she may minimize and even trivialize the client's experience of the problem (Nylund & Corsiglia, 1994).

Solution-focused therapy is an effective method of short-term treatment, however, it is one-sided and its lens is one of either/or rather than one of both/and. As in the previous models of problem-focused theories, half of the client is out of the picture. It is important to broaden the therapy lens to include all aspects that the client brings in to session and to honor each equally. People suffering from a chronic illness go unheard by many others, this feeling of invalidation can lower feelings of already jarred self-worth and perpetuate symptoms of the illness.

Complexity of Chronic Illness

The Problem with Certainty

"To know" something seems something to be taken for granted and can be assumed will occur. In today's world, however, this is not so. A universal reality cannot exist because of the many perceptions of any one particular event. What this means is that a person's story of the world and how it works is not the world, it is our interpretation of these constructions (Atwood, 1996). The difficulty is that many of the beliefs and attitudes a person holds were chosen for him or her, not by him or her (Salt & Neimark, 2002). This worldview taken into the realm of therapy offers the client a long overdue opportunity to offer his or her views regarding the problems he or she walks in with.

As a therapist, this may seem difficult to comprehend, questions such as, "what good will I do in a therapeutic setting if I do not have the answers for my clients?" This lens of therapy does not take away from the competence of the therapist, but rather it enhances the competencies of the client. When therapists dethrone themselves, a space is created for the client to become experts on their own issues (Duncan, Hubble, & Miller, 1997). This focuses on the client's strengths without ignoring the presenting problem. Learning the client's theory means taking the time to explore the client's thoughts, feelings, and attitudes about the nature of the problem (Duncan, Hubble, & Miller, Networker Conference, 1998; Salt & Neimark, 2002). Part of this procedure also involves exploring how the client might handle his or her current problem.

Change that occurs within the therapy room is only modestly correlated with technical wizardry and not at all correlated with any particular therapeutic school. It is far more heavily influenced by what clients bring into the room and the relationship that is created there (Duncan, Miller, & Hubble, 1997). The client's reality is respected and taken as such ... his or her own reality. This ownership of one's reality can be deeply disturbed when the crisis of searching for concrete answers around a chronic illness arises.

The Crisis

A chronic illness may be so disturbing to an individual as to cause a crisis within him or her. A sufferer of IBS may experience feelings of loss of control, shame, embarrassment, or guilt due to the lifestyle change that occurs when dealing with IBS symptoms. The symptoms are not only painful and unpleasant but also embarrassing and occur at inopportune moments (Salt & Neimark, 2002). The boundary experience of a crisis separates the individual from others in his or her interactive community and requires new boundary setting to include the illness (McNamee, 1992). These new boundaries will serve to provide a frame for the person to then develop a story around his or her reality. This story will provide a meaningful frame for a lived experience (Epston, White, & Murray, 1992).

In Western society, concrete evidence, facts, and observable realities rule how society views events. In a chronic illness such as IBS, these things do not exist. There is no test to take to discover evidence of the illness and no way to scientifically prove the diagnosis other than the reporting of symptoms by the patient. In a society where truth is coveted and held in highest importance, IBS can cause serious conflict within an individual, his or her family, and the medical setting in which they find themselves. The crisis that occurs may be defined as a decentralized identity and the IBS sufferer may experience himself or herself as having limited choices for a life story; going back to complete healthiness, or slipping fully into an unhealthy domain (McNamee, 1992). This is the either/or view once again. Through a more integrative approach the client can experience and appreciate the both/and lens of a post modern view.

The Biopsychosocial Model

The integration of the biological, psychological, and sociological aspects of dealing with a chronic illness allow the client to fully understand the issues surrounding his or her ongoing symptoms. This multi-factored perspective suggests an interaction of these three aspects of a person's life and that these aspects are determinants of his or her health, the onset of symptoms, and often the prognosis (Atwood, 1997). IBS symptoms have been linked to psychological stress and often increase during periods of such stress. Factors such as cognition, emotion, and motivation for behavior and mental processes contribute to a person's proneness for illness and also his or her speed of recovery (Atwood, 1997; Rolland, 1994). The mind, body, and spirit act together as a system and a disturbance in one causes a disturbance in the other two (Drossman, 2001). These factors are socially constructed because of the very nature of one's being ... we are social creatures and all that is taken in is processed in ways conducive to a particular belief system.

The belief system will influence largely how a person will react to his or her chronic illness. This system has been constructed by family/societal values, lifestyles, and previous experience with illness (Atwood, 1997). The individual needs to understand how these belief systems are affecting the symptoms of his or her illness. This understanding can create boundaries with the chronic illness included in the story of life rather than the illness demanding the main part. If these boundaries are not established and maintained, illness can invade the entire family system and the family will become uni-focused on the illness (Atwood, 1997).

The therapeutic lens of this model encourages the client, it empowers him or her about future possibilities, future choices, and future stories around which to base his or her life (Rolland, 1994). These narratives are based on empowerment rather than shame and the client learns how to rewrite caregiving scripts, and to encourage intimacy and maximize autonomy for all family members (Rolland, 1994). The process whereby therapists, clients, and the community develop critical consciousness is the first and necessary step toward empowerment and accountability (Hernandez, et al, 2005). This model offers a sense of self and ownership in a world where chronic illness can easily rob these precious commodities. The implication of this is that achieving health is an active process—in which you must participate fully—rather than a passive one in which some drug, pill, or treatment will cure you (Salt & Neimark, 2002).

Living with Uncertainty

Social Constructionism

Social constructionism is a worldview that involves a both/and perspective. In other words, one must view life events and interpretations as just that—interpretations. These perspectives have been brought about by belief systems that are in place because of the very events that are occurring. Language is the means by which these belief systems and scripts for life are transferred from one generation to the next. Built in to these narratives are the scripts that will determine what social stimuli a person internalizes and what is discarded. The process of raising critical consciousness presupposes that when we transform in ourselves, we simultaneously transform our relationship with others and the community that embraces us (Martin Baro, 1994).

In chronic illnesses these scripts determine the individual and family reaction to the crisis of such an identity change. Scripts operate at social, personal, and intrapsychic levels (Atwood, 1996) and each of these levels are disturbed with chronic illness. IBS affects a person's self-esteem, it also affects close interpersonal and social relationships because of the social isolation that may exist. What you choose to believe about IBS is critical, it will dramatically influence your attitude and the strength of conviction to practice behaviors to overcome IBS (Salt & Neimark, 2002). How an individual feels toward his or her chronic illness and the language he or she uses can perpetuate a set of beliefs about the illness. If particular forms of conversation can sustain identities, belief systems, and lines of action than it is possible that conversations and significant interactions can provide the opportunity for defining the crisis thereby redefining boundaries (McNamee, 1992). Language provides the means of both definition and redefinition.

Narratives between therapist and client provide the seeds of change. With an understanding of how beliefs have been constructed, these beliefs can then be deconstructed and then reconstructed according to the client's needs and wants. This collaborative approach creates mindful attitudes that enables the therapist to revisit pressures to dehumanize the experience of the illness and reduce the person and family system to a diseased patient and/or disorder (Rolland & Walsh, 2005). The transformational power of narrative rests in its capacity to re-relate the events of our client's lives in the context of new and different meaning (Anderson & Goolishian, 1992). Our lives are socially constructed through language, it follows that in order to promote change/growth, we must do so in the same realm. In a society built on absolute truth, knowledge, and reality, it is disconcerting to be on such slippery, uncertain ground. Acceptance leads not to surrender but to serenity, not to fear but to freedom, (Salt & Neimark, 2002). We must learn to embrace the unknown and accept the notion of truth as a "multiversal" truth rather than a universal one.

Narrative Considerations

Narrative therapy provides the client a forum in which to discuss these issues of social construction and come to an understanding of how these events have affected his or her current reaction to chronic illness. The overriding, dominant scripts are the ones that receive the most attention because of their primacy and potency among people's options (Atwood, 1996). These are the scripts that demand the most attention because of cultural, gender, or ethnic persuasions. These can become the problem-dominated narratives in times of crisis or identity transitions, such as a chronic illness. The narrative approach helps clients move from being influenced by these problem-dominated stories to more preferred stories (Zimmerman & Dickerson, 1994). The dominant scripts do not often include options for change or boundary flexibility. Creating appropriate boundaries allows you to become the master of your destiny—freeing you from the bondage of needing other people's approval (Cloud & Townsend, 1992). The narratives are created by people seeking to make meaning out of "deviations" from what their culture considers normal or ordinary (White, Epston, & Murray, 1992; Zimmeran & Dickerson, 1994; Atwood, 1996). Through the gradual decoding of their world, people can grasp the mechanisms of oppression and dehumanization of others—critical consciousness of others and of the surrounding reality brings with it the possibility of new forms of consciousness (Martin Baro, 1994). By exploring these topics the client's options are greatly increased.

Narrative metaphors increase understanding and options of both the individual response and also the response of family. A narrative metaphor would include the notion of pattern but extend it by looking at the meaning each member made of the other's response and to the effects of that response and them and the relationship (Nicholson, 1994; Zimmerman, & Dickerson, 1994). The therapist looks for the effect that IBS has on each family member involved and asks how has that person storied this event, when have the exceptions to his or her dominant stories occurred, and what are the possibilities for a different view in the future?

An initial step to re-storying is to externalize the illness from the family so that the family maintains its identity. By externalizing IBS from the family system, they can feel as a whole system and not as a "system of illness." In other words, the family maintains its sense of family self in the face of an identity crisis. Using externalizing language, separating client from illness and bringing forth future stories often has the effect of deconstructing both stories and leaving room for other experiences that have not emerged up until this time (Zimmerman & Dickerson, 1994). The therapist looks for times of healthy stories in the client's repertoire, he or she builds on exceptions that have occurred where shame and embarrassment were not the overriding factors in making decisions or responses to particular decisions. By looking for exceptions that are not currently being storied, those which do not fit into the dominant narrative, questions can be asked to recognize these alternatives and develop them more fully.

The Book of Life

Re-storying a life of chronic illness provides the client with a feeling of triumph, control, and power over an illness that possibly took over his or her life at one time. Finding alternatives already existing within the Book of Life makes this constructed reality easier to accept as one's own. The possibility of shifting and redefining boundaries becomes possible when clients cooperatively negotiate the need for such redefinition (McNamee, 1992). The dialogical process that occurs in the therapy assists the client in placing the illness in an externalized area and regaining power over his or her life. IBS sufferers learn they are more than an illness and that the mind-body connection is very real. Narrative therapy offers them validation of their feelings of shame and embarrassment while simultaneously focusing on their strengths and exceptions—truly a both/and experience.

The therapeutic conversation stimulates possibilities for the client because the therapist accepts the position of uncertainty involved in the socially-constructed world. Because he or she is in the position of "not knowing," a collaborative effort exists between client and therapist to generate these new meanings based in language (Anderson & Goolishian, 1992). There is an opening for the client, so that he or she is the expert on his or her reality, and is able to make changes and create new possibilities.

Possibilities

The crisis of a chronic illness brings about a world of many unknowns and shakes the foundation of an individual. He or she then seeks therapy to deal with this issue and is told there is no true reality, nothing is certain, and nothing can be truly known. The guidance of the therapist is vitally important in this area, he or she must delicately introduce these ideas after a validation of the person's presenting problem. When delicately placed, these notions can have a very calming effect on a client because they bring about possibilities. A crisis becomes a wonderful moment, to free oneself from ideas of "correctness," "objectivity," and "acceptance" and redesign or reconstruct one's place in the ongoing narrative of his or her life story (McNamee, 1992). The knowledge that there are exceptions, chances, and choices creates a very different world for these individuals.

The stance of the therapist is also important in narrative therapies. A position of "not knowing" or of curiosity provides the opportunity for the construction of new forms of action and interpretation (Cecchin, 1992). This approach is simple in its view and respects the client's authority on his or her life. The emphasis is not to produce change but to open space for conversations. Change in this therapy is represented by a dialogical creation of new narratives (Anderson & Goolishian, 1992). As the dialogue develops new stories are mutually created. We should always attempt to deconstruct our world as we know it, looking for the unexpected that might replace that view (Lax, 1992). Create an opening and new possibilities will arise.

These new possibilities have always been present but because of firmly-constructed scripts have not previously been noticed. Shadow scripts are connected to an individual's dominant scripts because they are composed of the opposite, of what is not said, and behaviors not acted out (Atwood, 1996). These are the scripts emphasized in narrative therapy and these provide the client with a sense of self-worth because they themselves held these scripts but were not actively pursuing them.

Making Peace with Uncertainty

The both/and lens or worldview carries with it the element of uncertainty. For western society this is a leap of faith and a difficult view to attain. Maintaining the position of "not knowing" requires that the therapist's understandings, explanations, and interpretations in therapy not be limited to his or her own constructed truths (Anderson & Goolishian, 1992). The therapist must accept the both/and lens as a *worldview* not only a means to a therapeutic end.

The both/and view involves faith in the unknown and uncertainty in the universe, it demands a broader, all-encompassing perspective of life. Western psychology has dealt poorly with the spiritual side of nature, not accepting things on faith but rather consistently demanding empirical data. In so doing, it has chosen to ignore human nature or has labeled it as pathological (Atwood & Maltin, 1991). In IBS, acceptance encourages you to make peace with your limitations at the same time it encourages you to seek out new treatment options to help you reduce your pain (Salt & Neimark, 2002). With the introduction and understanding of the Uncertainty Principle (Heisenberg, 1927), links between western society and a more philosophical eastern approach are necessary. The study of quantum physics suggests that it is impossible to measure a particle on the quantum level because to do so disturbs the system and, depending on the view of the physicist, the element could be a particle or a wave. This is disconcerting information for those entrenched in empirical data and freeing for those hoping for a more global approach.

For the chronically ill, particularly IBS sufferers, alternative medicines may provide for relief of symptoms. Eastern views of medicine encompass a both/and approach and work with an element of uncertainty on a daily basis. There are not scientifically-proven reasons for why many of the Eastern approaches work but many people, including Westerners, use these alternative forms in addition to Western/modern medicine. Alternative medicine is a trend driven largely by consumers (Westerners), particularly those with chronic illnesses who say they find relief in such treatments (Eisenberg, 1998). Perhaps the chronically-ill person is fed up with being treated like a malfunctioning body part and not a whole person (Markowitz, 1996).

Dealing with uncertainty creates an atmosphere of vulnerability, an unknowing, unsure approach to all things in life—nothing can be concretely explained or be an absolute truth. Eastern philosophy describes basic vulnerability as the seed of enlightenment already in us (Atwood & Maltin, 1991). With vulnerability comes power. The ability to perceive good and bad, black and white, and right and wrong allows you to develop a spiritual maturity with which to confront life's difficulties (Salt & Neimark, 2002). Our society cannot yet comprehend that strength can be represented by a leap of faith and a belief in uncertainty.

It is said that when this seed of enlightenment is freed and nurtured, it becomes the tender heart and in all its power can cut through barriers that all human beings seem to create (Atwood & Maltin, 1991).

Writer's Commentary

In preparing this chapter, the author learned to appreciate the greater scheme of accepting into one's life a both/ and view and allowing for uncertainty to be a factor in daily living. Although difficult to deal with, uncertainty brings with it a sense of relief because to know that all cannot be controlled is a breath of fresh air for all of those who attempt to control all.

In caring for the chronically ill, it is important to introduce uncertainty slowly because of the amount of uncertainty already enveloping their lives. It may or may not be a sense of comfort initially, but certainly a broadened perspective, a knowledge of choices, and a faith in themselves will ease the struggle of a new life ahead.

References

Aggarwal, V., McBeth, J., Zakrzewska, J., Lunt, M., & Macfarlane, G. (2006). The epidemiology of chronic syndromes that are frequently unexplained: do they have common associated factors? *International Journal of Epidemiology*, 35, 468-476.

Andersen, H. & Goolishian, H. (1992). The client is the expert: A not knowing approach. Chapter in *Therapy as Social Construction*, p. 25-40 (Gergen & McNamee, Eds.). Sage: Thousand Oaks, California.

Atwood, J (1996). *Family Scripts*. Basic Books: New York.

Atwood, J. (1997). *Family Systems, Family Medicine: A Collaboration in Dialogue*. Internet publication.

Atwood, J. & Maltin, L. (1991). Putting eastern philosophy in western psychotherapy. *American Journal of Psychotherapy*, 55, 368-382.

Bartunek, K. & Mock, M. (1994). First order, second order, and third order change and organizational development intervention: a cognitive approach. *Journal of Applied Sciences*, 23, 483-500.

Beavers, W. R. & Hampson, R. B. (1993). Measuring family competence. In *Normal Family Processes*, 2nd edition, Walsh, F. (Ed). Guilford: New York.

Beavers, W. & Voeller, M. (1983). Family models: Comparing and contrasting the Olson circumplex model with the Beavers system model. *Family Process*, 22, 85-98.

Ben-David, A. & Jurich, J. (1993). A Test of Adaptability: Examining the curvilinear assumption. *Journal of Family Psychology*, 7, 370-375.

Boss, P. (2001). *Family Stress Management*. Sage: Newbury Park, CA.

Burg, M. & Seeman, T. (1994). Families and health: The negative side of social ties. *Annals of Behavioral Medicine*, 16, 109-115.

Campbell, T. (2003). The effectiveness of family interventions for physical disorders. *Journal of Marital and Family Therapy*, April, 263-282.

Christiansen, C. (2001). Wellness, health and happiness, a complicated combination. *Women's Health Weekly*, December 13, 2001.

DeShazer, S. (1991). *Putting Difference to Work*. W.W. Norton: New York.

Donoghue, D. & Siegel, M. (1992). *Sick and Tired of Feeling Sick and Tired*. W.W. Norton: New York.

Duncan, B., Hubble, M., & Miller, S. (1997). Stepping off the throne. *Family Therapy Networker*, July-August, 22-33.

Eisenberg, C. (1998). Medical marriage. *Newsday*, May 6, 1998.

Falvo, D. (1991). *Medical and Psychosocial Aspects of Chronic Illness and Disability*. Aspen: Gaithersburg, MD.

George, L. K. & Gwyther, L. P. (1986). Caregiver wellbeing: A mulimensional examination of family caregivers of demented adults. *The Gerontologist*, 26, 253-259.

Gilligan, C. (1982). *In a Different Voice: Psychological Theory and Women's Development.* Harvard University Press: Cambridge, MA.

Hamilton, G. (1989). A critical review of object relations theory. *American Journal of Psychiatry,* 12, 1552-1559.

Hardy, K. (1993). Live supervision in the post modern era of family therapy: Issues, reflections and questions. *Contemporary Family Therapy,* 15, 9-20.

Heisenberg (1927). *Uncertainty Principle.* Internet Publication. *http://www.ispn.com/njurick/werner.html.*

Hernandez, P., Almeida, A., & Dolan Del-Vecchio, K. (2005). Critical consciousness, accountability, and empowerment: Key process for helping families heal. *Family Process,* March, 105-120.

Hill, R. (1958). Generic features of families under stress. *Social Casework,* 49, 139-150.

Kerns, R. & Weiss, L. (1994). Family influence on the course of chronic illness: a cognitive behavioral transaction model. *Annals of Behavioral Medicine,* 16, 116-121.

Kowal, J., Johnson, S., & Lee, A. (2003). Chronic illness in couples: A case for emotionally focused therapy. *Journal of Marital and Family Therapy,* 29, 299.

Livneh, H. & Antonak, R. (2005). Psychosocial adaptation to chronic illness: A primer for counselors. *Journal of Counseling and Development,* 83, 12-20.

Luthar, S. S., Cicchetti, D., & Becker, B. (2000). The construct of resilience: A critical evaluation and guidelines for future work. *Child Development,* 71, 543-562.

Madigan, S. (1992). The application of Michael Foucault's philosophy in problem externalizing discourse of Michael White. *Journal of Family Therapy,* 14, 265-279.

Markowitz, L. (1996). Minding the body, embodying the mind. *Family Therapy Networker,* September/October, 22-26.

Marks, N., Lambert, J.d., & Choi, H. (2002). Transitions in caregiving, gender, and psychological well-being: A Prospective U.S. national study. *Journal of Marriage and Family,* 64, 657-668.

Martin-Baro, I. (1994). *Writings for a Liberation Psychology.* Harvard University Press: Cambridge, MA.

McCubbin et al, (1980). Developing family vulnerability to stress: Coping patterns and strategies wives employ. In J. Trost (Ed.) *The Family and Change,* pages 89-103. International Library: Sweden.

McCubbin, H, McCubbin, M., & Thompson, E. (1995). Resiliency in Ethnic families: A conceptual model for predicting family adjustment and adaptation. In H. McCubbin, M. McCubbin, A. Thompson, & J. Fromer (Eds). *Resiliency in Ethnic Minority Families.* (Vol. 1, pages 3-48). Madison, WI: University of Wisconsin Press.

McCubbin, H. & Patterson, J. (1983). The family stress process: The double ABCX model of family adjustment and adaptation. *Marriage and Family Review,* 61 (1-2), 7-37.

Minuchin, S. (1975). A conceptual model of psychosomatic illness in children: Family organization and family therapy. *Archives of General Psychiatry,* 32, 1031-1038.

Moos, R. H. (1988). Psychosocial factors in the work place. Chapter in *Handbook of Life Stress,* 344, (Fisher, S. & Reason, J., Eds.). Wiley and Sons: Portsmouth, U.K.

Nicholson, S. (1995) The narrative dance: A practice map for Michael White's therapy. *Australian and New Zealand Journal of Family Therapy,* 16, 23-28.

Nylund, D. & Corsiglia, N. (1994). Becoming solution-focused forced in brief therapy: Remembering something important we already knew. *Journal of Systemic Therapy,* 13, 5-11.

Olson, D. H., Portner, J. & Lavee, Y. (1985). FACES III, University of Minnesota.

Olson, D. H., Russell, C. S., & Sprenkle, D. H. (1989). Circumplex Model of Marital and Family Systems. Haworth Press: Binghamton, NY.

Patterson, J. & Garwick, A. (1994). The impact of chronic illness on families: A family systems perspective. *Annals of Behavioral Medicine*, 16, 131-142.

Patterson, J. (1988). Families experiencing stress: The family adjustment and adaptation response model. *Family Systems Medicine*, 5(2), 202-237.

Rampage, C. (1994). Power, gender, and marital intimacy. *Journal of Family Therapy*, 16, 125-137.

Register, C. (1987). *Living with Chronic Illness: Days of Patience and Passion.* The Free Press: New York.

Revenson, T. (1994). Social support and marital coping with chronic illness. *Annals of Behavioral Medicine*, 16, 122-130.

Rice, P. (1992). *Stress and Health.* Brooks/Cole: Belmont, CA.

Rolland, J. (1989). Chronic illness and the family life cycle. Chapter in *The Changing Family Life Cycle: A Framework for Family Therapy*, 433-457, (Carter, B. & McGoldrick, B., Eds.). Allyn & Bacon: Boston.

Rolland, J. (1994). *Families, Illness and Disability: An Integrative Treatment Model.* Basic Books: New York.

Rolland, J. & Walsh, F. (2005). Systemic training for healthcare professionals: The Chicago Center for Family health approach. *Family Process*, 44, 283-302.

Rolland, J. & Williams, J. (2005). Toward a biopsychosocial model for 21st century genetics. *Family Process*, 44, 3-25.

Salt, W. (1995). *Irritable Bowel Syndrome and the Mind-Body/Brain Gut Connection.* Haworth: Boston.

Schmaling, K. B., & Sher, T. G. Eds. (2000). *The Psychology of Couples and Illness: Theory, Research, and Practice.* American Psychological Association: Washington, DC.

Schwartz, L., Slater, M. A., & Birchler, G. R. (1996) The role of pain behaviors in the modulation of marital conflict in chronic pain couples. *Pain*, 65, 227-233.

Seltzer, M. M. & Li, L.W. (2000). The dynamics of caregiving: Transitions during a three year prospective study. *The Gerontologist*, 40, 107-116.

Snyder, K. D., Cavell, T. A., Heffer, R. W., & Mangrum, L. F. (1995). "Marital and family assessment: A multifaceted, multilevel approach." In *Integrating Family Therapy: Handbook of Family Psychology and Systems Theory*, Mikesell, R.H.; Lusterman, D.D.; McDaniel, S.H. (Eds.) American Psychological Association: Washington, DC.

Towns, A. (1994). Asthma, power and the therapeutic conversation. *Family Process*, 33, 161-174.

Trepper, T., Dolan, Y., McCollum, E., & Nelson, T. (2006). Steve deShazer and the future of solution focused therapy. *Journal of Marital and Family Therapy*, 32, 133-140.

Walsh, F. (1998). *Strengthening Family Resilience.* Guilford Press: New York

Walsh, F. (2003). Family resilience: A framework for clinical practice. *Family Process*, 42. 18.

Wilday, S. & Dovey, A. (2005). All in the mind? *Occupational Health*, 57, 25-29.

Wilkinson, D. (2003). Among the ailments symptoms: Acute embarrassment. *New York Times*, June 22, 2003.

Young, R. F. & Kahana, E. (1989). Specifying caregiver outcomes: Gender and relationship aspects of caregiving strain. *The Gerontologist*, 29, 660-666.

Zimmerman, J. & Dickerson, V. (1994). Using a narrative metaphor: Implications for theory and clinical practice. *Family Process*, 33, 233-245.

7

A Family Case Study on Mindfulness-Based Family Therapy for Chronic Co-Occurring Disorders: Chronic Stress, Chronic Anxiety, and Chronic Pain

Anthony R. Quintiliani

Abstract

Advances in mindfulness-based clinical research in the past decade have increased dramatically. Mindfulness-based therapies include such areas as stress reduction, breathing therapy, cognitive therapy and extensions of cognitive-behavioral therapy. One area that has not received much attention is the application of mindfulness-based interventions to family therapy. This article will be an attempt to remedy that problem.

Family Therapy Model

This chapter represents a new integration of more traditional family therapy orientations (strategic, structural, systemic, and cognitive-behavioral) with the important approach of mindfulness-based family therapy. This new family therapy integration uses more typical family therapy processes to teach and practice mindfulness-based skills designed to reduce chronic stress, anxiety, depression, substance abuse, chronic pain, and other areas of family dysfunction.

Of all the traditional family therapy approaches used with this family, perhaps cognitive-behavioral family therapy is the best fit for what transpired. Mindfulness-based family therapy decreases systemic risk factors in chronic conditions, enhances family-based coping skills, develops parental mindfulness capacities, and strengthens interpersonal interactions within the family system (Hayes, Follette, & Linehan, 2004; Woodberry, et al, 2002; Miller, et al, 2002; Dumas, 2005).

Mindfulness-based family therapy includes family skill areas of stress reduction, breathing therapy, cognitive therapy, meditation, and extensions of cognitive-behavioral therapy. This family case study on family therapy of chronic conditions is an attempt to present such a formulation. This chapter will also clarify what aspects of more traditional family therapy approaches were used with the family. The main theme is to clarify how to use mindfulness-based family therapy as treatment of chronic clinical conditions within a family.

Definition of Chronic Illness

Chronic clinical illness includes many of the most common and difficult problems to treat in clinical practice. Some characteristics of chronic conditions are progressive deterioration, more or less permanent impairments, severe and prolonged suffering, and sometimes fatal outcomes. The three chronic conditions dealt with in this chapter are chronic systemic family stress, chronic anxiety, and chronic pain. In the family therapy of behavioral health, the most common chronic conditions include combinations of substance use, anxiety, resistant depression, obesity, severe and persistent mental illness, systemic stress, and comorbid medical conditions.

Purpose of this Chapter

This chapter is an attempt to close the current deficit in mindfulness-based clinical interventions within family therapy. The main focus here is to present "how to" include mindfulness-based interventions in a family therapy treatment episode.

Since these mindfulness-based family interventions represent the core of this chapter, far less information about more typical family therapy models will be presented. Furthermore, many of the mindfulness-based interventions will be presented with sufficient detail to enable informed family therapists to practice these skills within their family therapy of choice.

Gaps in Current Family Therapy Research and Practice

Although there are many, many available references in research and practice literature about various forms of family therapy, there exists a serious dearth of articles and books dealing with mindfulness-based family therapy. The clinical bibliography published by The Center for Mindfulness in Meditation, Health Care, and Society in Springfield, Massachusetts lists over seventy-five references, most of which refer to evidence-based research and practice. Not a single reference covers the use of mindfulness-based family therapy. *The Journal of Marital and Family Therapy*, 33(4) includes six articles on the topic.

Summary of Mindfulness-Based Family Therapy

Referral Conditions and Background

The family presented in this chapter has been disguised to protect confidentiality, and some of the mindfulness-based clinical interventions have been masked to prevent accidental identification. Furthermore, some of the family therapy interventions noted are of a composite nature—not solely used with this family. All of this has been done to protect privacy.

The Primary Care Physician's Role

The physician who collaborated in this case of mindfulness-based family therapy played several important roles. The physician made an initial rule-out screening of behavioral health conditions that required follow-up by a psychologist. Following her physician's recommendation, the client pursued more formal behavioral health assessment. The client and her family continued to receive routine medical care from their physician. The physician also monitored the related medical needs of family members, as well as various medications issues. Without the informed and motivated attention of her physician, the client and her family might not have received the necessary clinical interventions for their various clinical conditions. The physician's on-going support to continue family therapy was another important determinant of outcomes.

The family suffered from severe anxiety-related conditions. The mother experienced generalized anxiety and anxiety-induced overeating; the father (a partner) suffered from chronic pain and fearful apprehension about his ability to function at work on a daily basis; and, the son had enduring attention deficit disorder without hyperactivity. The family system experienced long-term chronic stress, which interacted with and exacerbated all their existing chronic problems.

The mother (I will refer to her as Joan) presented as the identified client initially. She presented with features of generalized anxiety disorder comorbid with symptoms of anxiety-induced eating behaviors, mild depression, and alcohol abuse. However, once more in-depth assessment was completed, it became evident that her comorbidity was less severe and that a family therapy intervention would be more appropriate for all three family members. This possibility was especially attractive to the therapist and the family because it allowed great efficiency in the number of sessions required and thus reduced financial burdens for the family. Since the family had limited insurance coverage and inconsistent weekly income, all members of the family agreed to participate in family sessions.

During the assessment phase of family therapy, it became apparent that this family had suffered from long-term chronic stress and low socioeconomic status. Both parents had not graduated from high school and were employed in relatively low-paying jobs. Financial strain was the most common source of parental conflict and family pressure.

Joan completed her GED, worked part time and attended some business classes at a local junior college; she expressed hope that additional education might improve her employment possibilities. Such a schedule, however, meant that the family's more traditional roles, rules, and expectations were simply added to her already stressful life. By the end of the day she often found herself exhausted, alienated, and sometimes quick-tempered. When she became emotionally upset she would often isolate herself and eat as a way to self-soothe and relax.

This was a traditional family structure; however, the parents never made their marriage official. Work stress, emotional overload, and sympathetic nervous system arousal often led to emotional conflict between the parents. Usually the sources of such conflicts were stressors and misunderstandings in the home, unpaid bills, and unwillingness by the father ("after a hard day in construction work") to help out at home.

Matthew (not his real name) was Joan's long-term partner. After dropping out of high school, he obtained a construction job; with hard work he was able to obtain a training position in house framing and interior finish work. He was a hard-working man, who appeared dedicated to Joan and her son. His job provided a reasonable but highly inconsistent weekly income for the family. Matthew suffered from a work-related back injury that left him with mild-to-moderate chronic low back pain. The injury was not severe enough to impair his employability; however, after longer days of physically demanding work, he sometimes experienced moderate-to-severe pain. He reported that although his back pain never abated on most days he could tolerate it. When he was tired and when his back pain was "acting up" he experienced low frustration tolerance, sometimes resulting in emotional reactivity, social isolation, and irritability. He also experienced some guilt and concern about whether he could in his words "be a good provider for his family."

Chris (a pseudonym) was Joan's 13 year-old son from a previous long-term relationship. He also suffered from an anxiety-related clinical condition—attention deficit disorder without hyperactivity or ADD. He was born out of wedlock when Joan was much younger; his biological father deserted the family shortly after the birth. The son of a loving, low socioeconomic status, single-parent, Chris was well aware of his learning problems and his relative poverty. He also suffered from low self-esteem. When his parents argued and isolated from each other, or when their own clinical conditions were activated, Chris found himself preoccupied, lonely, despaired, and fearful. It was quite clear that his ADD caused learning problems at school, and it was also clear that parental conflict, chronic family stress, and limited financial means impaired his ability to function and develop as a more typical young adolescent.

Diagnostic Implications, Treatment Targets and a Mindfulness-Based Family Therapy Approach

Various mindfulness-based family therapy assessments and interventions are noted below. Since Joan suffered from more problems, she received a more complete assessment. The Beck Depression Inventory, the Beck Anxiety inventory, the CAGE Alcohol Screening, the Short Michigan Alcoholism Screening Test, and various diagnostic interviews on major symptoms were completed. Since the only positive screens indicated problems with anxiety and overeating (which did not meet clinical criteria for an eating disorder), a clinical interview for generalized anxiety disorder was included. The anxiety-induced overeating remained a clinical target because her slow weight gain over time was sometimes a source of conflict with Matthew. Also, parental behavioral patterns of isolating in negative emotional moods made family interactions problematic and reinforced family stress, eating problem and family dysfunction.

Other family members did not appear to present as many clinical problems. Matthew had already received a medical work-up for his chronic pain condition, and he was well aware of his apprehension about remaining employed with his limitations. His mindfulness-based family therapy clinical targets were chronic pain and improved interactional patterns with others. Due to earlier school related assessments Chris had a very clear mindfulness target—to learn to improve his focus and attention. All family members needed to improve their emotional responses to chronic stress and interactional patterns; systemic and interpersonal stressors exacerbated already existing anxiety and pain conditions.

It was reasonably clear that this family's clinical conditions would benefit from mindfulness-based family therapy. Psychoeducation included ways that mindfulness training could be helpful to the family. The following mindfulness-based stress reduction interventions were included in treatment.

Mindfulness-based breathing therapy and various ways to use the breath helped to stabilize sympathetic nervous system arousal and emotional/fear responses in the limbic system. Body-scanning techniques located and altered bodily locations of tension as well as modified pain perception. Vipassana meditation techniques (Hart, 1987; Marlatt, 2004) were helpful in detecting cognitive and physical cues leading to incidents of emotional reactivity. Other whole-family ritualized mini-meditation practices (candle gazing, listening to soothing sounds, etc.) slowly conditioned family members away from anxious appraisal, isolation, counterproductive alliances and toward family integration with calming expectations. These practices and skills improved family cohesion.

The family's chronic stress was pervasive. Chronic clinical problems and conflictual interactions often led to a chaotic family structure. Emotional distance was regulated via discrete boundaries, and attachment was regulated via enmeshment. The family history and emotional patterns implied that the mother and son became more enmeshed over time, as the mother and father became more distant over time. Themes and interaction behaviors may have been used to titrate stress tolerance and emotional regulation within the system (Lewis, 1986; Figley & McCubbin, 1983).

Related Family Therapy Awareness

From structural family therapy, boundaries were used to clarify subsystem interactions versus whole family interactions. Systemic rules, roles, and demands were clarified. Rather than the parents excluding Chris from serious family discussions, he was now included in family problem solving and in family meditations. When family enactments began in sessions, mindfulness-based family therapy skills were used to restructure family rigidity into more flexible understandings and behaviors. Since Joan and Chris had stronger emotional ties, psychoeducation was provided to help them reduce coalition behaviors that might alienate Matthew. Since both parents hoped to exclude Chris from their conflicts, using alliance and coalition constructs helped to inform them about ways to expand whole family interactions without conflict. Changes implemented in mindfulness-based family therapy helped to change repetitive sequences of behavior, thereby modifying rules, roles, and boundaries. The family could function as a whole in family sessions and at home when skills were practiced (Colapinto, 1991; Aponte & Van Deusen, 1991).

From a strategic family therapy perspective, reframing and relabeling of symptoms were used to alter emotional, stress-induced arousal and reactivity. Family conflicts were reinterpreted and reframed. The more family members reacted to each other, the stronger their concern and love for each other. By improving the ability of family members to use mindfulness reframing every time they perceived a build up of negative energy, the more apt they were to move toward calm abiding as a family. Relational and communication processes were also improved through relabeling and reframing (Madanes, 1981; Madanes, 1984).

Parents were taught and helped to use mindfulness awareness skills to monitor and modify negative interaction patterns. This improved the parental subsystem. Homework was assigned to practice general mindfulness skills and specialized skills to improve interactions (Madanes, 1984).

Practical family problem solving therapy was included within mindfulness-based family therapy. The chronic stress and negative interaction problems were identified and witnessed as chronic anxiety. These problems were operationalized via interactional patterns (who did what, when and how). The solution hypothesis was clarified as mindfulness-based family therapy skills. Homework, family life experience, and in-session reenactments were testing grounds (Haley, 1976; Kelly, 1983).

From a cognitive-behavioral family therapy approach, such interventions as psychoeducation, mindfulness communications training, operant problem solving, and thought-emotion diaries on mindfulness were used to improve emotional interactions. The family could also learn to give and receive rewards (reinforcers) for improved interactions, and they could track thoughts and emotions related to positive and negative interactions. Mindfulness-based family therapy also improved coping skills for all family members; stress reduction and self-calming skills empowered the family to be less reactive (Fallon, 1991; Freeman, et.al. 1989; Hayes, Follette & Linehan, 2004).

From a systemic family therapy viewpoint, the family was taught how to interpret the context of problems as interactions between people within circular causality. Reciprocal and contingent interactional responses created strong homeostasis within the family. Chronic clinical conditions led to crisis, in which with guidance the family system could be changed (i.e., deviation amplification). Creative problem solving was pushed. The concept of family empowerment was useful in improving systemic self-efficacy. The family was encouraged to use as many skills as possible on as many days of the week as possible. Changing the self-perceptions of the family from conflictual to integrated, and doing daily family mini-meditation sessions helped to ensure ongoing effectiveness. Doing more things together, and doing more things more effectively, empowered the family toward recovery (O'Hanlon & Weiner-Davis, 1989; Schultz, 1984).

Additional family concerns led to practical strategic problem solving. Due to limited insurance coverage and lower income, costly medications might not be a viable treatment option. Psychostimulants for ADD, selective serotonin reuptake inhibitors for anxiety, and various opiates for pain management might have been helpful to this family. The family was not poor enough to obtain assistance, but neither was it wealthy enough to afford medications. There were also concerns about the addiction potential in using opiates for pain. Psychosocial interventions were the primary approaches used.

How Mindfulness-Based Family Therapy Noted Here May Address the Existing Gaps in Practice

Delivery of Mindfulness-Based Family Therapy

After basic mindfulness-based family therapy psychoeducation had been completed, actual clinical interventions began. The focus of this chapter is on how to use mindfulness-based family therapy to address multiple, chronic problems in a typical family system. The primary goal to improve chronic stress reactivity and the related clinical conditions interacting with it was well-matched to the types of interventions used. When the problem mix is appropriate, and when family members agree to be treated as a family, mindfulness-based family therapy can serve as a potent form of intervention.

Specific Mindfulness-Based Interventions

The family was taught how to use breathing techniques to self-calm. There is ample research supporting the effectiveness of breathing retraining to reduce autonomic and limbic reactivity in various clinical conditions (Kabat-Zinn & Chapman-Waldrop, 1988; Hanh, T. N, 1990; Fried & Grimaldi, 1993; Kabat-Zinn, Chapman, & Salmon, 1997).

Breathing techniques such as slower diaphragmatic breathing, counting breaths, counting and visualizing breaths, extending exhalation, breathing into "the gap," breathing through the mouth, and more rapid deep breathing were used to teach family members how to achieve relaxation states. Homework was assigned for the whole family to practice breathing skills, and when possible to extend this into whole-family mini-meditation sessions (called "relaxation response" here). This allowed skill-practice to become a family ritual. Scheduled, daily practice sessions for short periods of time were encouraged strongly. Once family members could demonstrate that they could use these skills, the skills were used *invivo* in mindfulness-based family therapy sessions.

Invivo skills practice in sessions came up whenever family members began to escalate emotionally into typical cycles of conflict. Rather than simply observe, analyze, or intervene in such reenactments, I cued the family to practice here now what they had learned about reducing stress responses. In addition the family was taught how to measure and self-reinforce all skills practice. The self-measurement of anxiety and pain was accomplished by having family members use the Subjective Units of Disturbance Scale (SUDS—a Wolpe technique). Both anxiety and pain perception/sensitivity could be measured by using a SUDS from 1 to 10 or (as I prefer) from 1 to 100. Pre and post SUDS scores were used so subjective internal changes could be measured more objectively within the family. Family self-regulation of emotion, changes in SUDS scores, and daily skills practice increased the family's sense of empowerment.

Since so much clinical work has become negative and pathology-based, I developed a positively oriented scale like the SUDS. My own SUPS (Subjective Units of Pleasure Scale) was used with this family. Pre to post SUPS measures (from 1 to 100) were used to obtain more standardized measures of subjective improvements in emotion and pleasure. Use of pre to post SUPS documented improvements in patterns of negative interactions, again enhancing family-based empowerment to notice and improve happiness.

The ability of a family to use measures like SUDS in mindfulness-based family therapy to document reductions in perceived stress, anxiety, and pain is a step toward improved family empowerment and personal self-efficacy. The family members can measure improvements in emotion and mood with the SUPS. As the family worked toward improved coping capacities and skills via their own behaviors in mindfulness-based breathing, awareness, and meditation their sense of competence and confidence improved. I reminded the family often that there is no greater empowerment than to learn how to use the mind to better control both the brain and the body. The improvement of family-system consciousness can overcome some more hard-wired mind/body realities in anxiety and stress.

Another mindfulness-based intervention used with these family members was teaching them how to enhance positive memories and experiences by multi-modalization techniques. I introduced the family to multi-sensory information processing; when used in positive ways this intervention is the opposite of what happens in posttraumatic stress disorder flashbacks. Since we know the mind will automatically force multi-sensory memories on people suffering from severe PTSD, my technique uses cognitive intention to process sensory and memory inputs about positive experiences in multi-sensory ways. Acting "as if" the positive event can be reprocessed simply by intentionally using each sensory processing channel provided enhanced pleasure to this family. Positive family-related activities and any positive family memories can be reprocessed in this manner, thereby increasing time and energy in happier life experiences.

Instructions were easy to follow. Breathing calmly while sitting in a relaxed, quasi-meditative state each family member was asked to recall a pleasant substance-free experience. Once the cognitive memory was in place, each sensory processing channel was added: affective, behavioral, visual, auditory, kinesthetic, gustatory, olfactory, and spiritual. The SUPS was used in pre-to-post measures to document how adding more sensory processing channels enhanced the perceived quality of the experience. The more sensory processing channels used, the more brain cell firing in more parts of the brain. This brain-based change improved and strengthened the memory. Both self-efficacy regarding self-confidence (Bandura, 1997) and stress inoculation reinforcing self-talk (Meichenbaum, 1985) improved. Furthermore, such brain integration techniques within family therapy can improve cortical (frontal lobes, neo-cortex) inhibition over more reactive subcortical (autonomic and limbic) emotional reactions. Integration of responses can improve anxiety and family responses to chronic stress.

Family members were taught and practiced a wide range of mindfulness-based family therapy skills, including calm breathing, non-judgmental observation, body scanning, secular mini-meditations, etc. Such skills have been demonstrated in research and practice to improve anxiety, reduce obsessive worries, enhance emotional regulation, and reduce emotional distress (Linehan, 1993; Hanh, 1990; Kabat-Zinn, 2005; and, Kabat-Zinn, et al, 1992; Linehan, Bohus, & Lynch, 2007).

Another mindfulness-based family therapy skill included in this therapy episode was a simplified version of how to short-circuit sympathetic nervous system and limbic system stress reactions. Perhaps the single most important aspect of this family therapy intervention was to help family members recognize where the point of no return exists in stress responses. That is the place in a sequence of events where hard-wired neuro-anatomical stress pathways overpower the cortical (frontal, thinking, executive) brain. Psychophysiologic upheaval is the outcome; in such mind/body experiences, people cannot apply coping skills—their mind and body are now on automatic pilot and out of control.

My Tracking Back technique helped this family to recognize earlier and earlier stimuli/cues/red flags that eventually lead to full-blown stress reactions. Family members searched backwards for any event or awareness that presented into consciousness before the emotional reaction. Since powerful kinesthetic awareness of bodily signs implied it may be too late to prevent negative emotional reactions, locating earlier warning signs was helpful in maintaining some control over reactions to stressors. Once family members were able to recognize three earlier-in-sequence "pink flags," they were in a better position to apply specific mindfulness-based family stress reduction skills before negative emotions activated problematic patterns. Again, self-empowerment improved family functioning.

A few more mindfulness-based family therapy interventions were used with individual family members. These skills were taught in session and always recommended for home practice. Although some of the more typical skills (present moment awareness, mini-meditations, calming breath, and mentally disengaging from negative emotional events) helped with eating problems, a few more specific skills were needed. Joan learned to slowly focus attention and appreciation on her food; this form of multi-sensory awareness slowed down her generally rapid eating behaviors. She was also taught to eat smaller portions, to chew longer on smaller bites of food, etc. (Kristeller & Hallett, 1999; Kristeller, 2003).

Matthew, likewise, needed some additional skills for pain management. These included calm breathing when in pain, present moment awareness, mind/body relaxation, and muscular-skeletal tension reduction. Additional pain management techniques included lying meditation, gentle yoga stretches, calm intentional response to pain perception, mental distraction, paying attention to shifts in pain perception at the surrounding areas where pain existed, and anchoring all successful applications by touching a stone in his pocket (Kabat-Zinn, 1982; Kabat-Zinn, Lipworth, Burney, & Sellers, 1987).

Clinical Outcomes

After approximately fifteen sessions of MBFT over a five-month period, limited telephone coaching on skills practice, instructional handouts, homework, and in-office enactment practice the clinical objectives of this episode were more or less achieved. The core treatment goal of reducing chronic systemic stress in the family was highly successful. There appeared to be an interaction between family member skill development and the general level of reduced stress. Joan's anxiety and anxiety-induced over eating improved greatly; Matthew's pain tolerance improved, thereby improving his overall mood, expectations, and interpersonal interactions; and Chris showed minimal improvement in his ADD. Additionally, family members now possessed new mindfulness-based skills that improved family harmony and rituals. The family reported feeling more empowered to solve their own problems. Family rules, roles, boundaries, interactions, and empowerment all improved as a result of mindfulness-based family therapy. The use of SUDS and SUPS self-measures enhanced family empowerment to notice changes. There were no formal follow-ups with the family. The family was asked to recontact me if they again experienced chronic stress conditions, or if their individual problems flared up again. The family was given the option of having a three-to-six-month skills "tune-up" with me if desired.

Summary and Implications for Further Exploration

This chapter reviewed a successful application of mindfulness-based family therapy. Since so little has been published on using mindfulness-based interventions in family therapy, this brief chapter is simply a small beginning in addressing the existing dearth of research and practice literature on the topic. Clearly there exists great need to expand research and practice in mindfulness-based family therapy. This should occur more rapidly, since the proven effectiveness of both family therapy in general and mindfulness-based interventions for specific stress-related and biopsychosocial problems is quite strong in existing clinical literature.

More specific ways to generalize some of the implications of mindfulness-based family therapy are using mindfulness skills (as defined in family dialectical behavior therapy) to improve listening, validation, contingencies of reinforcement and commitments within family systems. Mindfulness about family safety, behavioral analysis, and crisis management skills may also improve emotional functioning of the entire family. Mindfulness also offers ways to strengthen parental capacities to be helpful and supportive. Parents are taught how to do facilitative listening so their responses will be nonjudgmental and more helpful. They also learn how to mindfully distance themselves from emotional dysregulated situations within the family. Parents and their children participate in motivational action plans (MAPs) to help solve their own family problems, thus allowing mindfulness skills to pave the way toward family empowerment (Miller, et.al 2002; Dumas, 2005). Additional research and practice in mindfulness in family therapy is needed.

References

American Psychiatric Association. (1994). *Diagnostic and Statistical Manual for Mental Disorders.* Vol. IV, Washington, DC: American Psychiatric Press.
Aponte, J. H. & Van Deusen, J. M. (1991). Structural family therapy. In A. Gurman & D. P. Kniskern (Eds.). *Handbook of Family Therapy,* Vol. 2, (pp. 310-360). New York: Brunner/Mazel.
Bandura, A. (1997). *Self-Efficacy: The Exercise of Control.* New York: W. W. Freeman.
Colapinto, J. (1991). Structural family therapy. In A. Gurman & D. P. Kniskern (Eds.). *Handbook of Family Therapy,* Vol. 2, (pp. 417-443). New York: Brunner/Mazel.
Dumas, J. E. (2005). Mindfulness-based parent training. *The Journal of Clinical Child and Adolescent Psychology,* 34(4), 779-791.
Fallon, I. R. H. (1991). Behavioral family therapy. In A. Gurman & D. P. Kniskern (Eds.). *Handbook of Family Therapy,* Vol. 2, (pp. 65-95). New York: Brunner/Mazel.
Freeman, A., Simon, K., & Beutler, L. et al, (1989). (Eds.). *Comprehensive Handbook of Cognitive Therapy.* New York: Plenum.
Haley, J. (1976). *Problem-Solving Therapy.* New York: Harper.
Hanh, T. N. (1990). *Present Moment, Wonderful Moment.* Berkeley, CA: Parallax.
Hart, W. (1987). *The Art of Living: Vipassana Meditation as Taught by S. N. Goenka.* San Francisco, CA: Harper Collins Publications.
Kabat-Zinn, J. (1982). An outpatient program in behavioral medicine for chronic pain patients based on the practice of mindfulness meditation. *General Hospital Psychiatry,* 4, 33-42.
Kabat-Zinn, J. (2005). *Coming to Our Senses: Healing Ourselves and the World Through Mindfulness.* New York: Hyperion.
Kabat-Zinn, J., Chapman-Waldrop, A. (1997). Compliance with an outpatient stress reduction program. *Journal of Behavioral Medicine,* 8, 333-352.
Kabat-Zinn, J., Chapman, A., & Salmon, P. (1997). The relationship of cognitive and somatic components of anxiety to patient preference for alternative relaxation techniques. *Mind Body Medicine,* 2, 101-109.
Kabat-Zinn, J., Lipworth, L., Burney, R., & Sellers, W. (1987). Four-year follow-up of a meditation-based program for the self-regulation of chronic pain. *Clinical Journal of Pain,* 2, 159-173.
Kabat-Zinn, J. et al (1992). Effectiveness of a meditation-based stress reduction program in the treatment of anxiety disorders. *American Journal of Psychiatry,* 149, 936-943.
Kelley, H. H. (1983). *Close Relationships.* New York: Freeman, pp. 436-442.
Kristeller, J. L. (2003). Mindfulness, wisdom and eating. *Journal of Constructivism in Human Services,* 8(2), 107-118.
Kristeller, J. L. & Hallett, C. B. (1999). An exploratory study of a mindfulness-based intervention for binge eating. *Health Psychology,* 4(3), 357-363.

Lewis, J. M. (1986). Family structure and stress. *Family Process*, 25(2), 235-247.

Linehan, M. M. (1993). *Skills Training Manual for Treating Borderline Personality Disorder.* New York: Guilford Publications, pp. 109-113.

Linehan, M. M., Bohus, M., & Lynch, T. R. (2007). Dialectical behavior therapy for pervasive emotional dysregulation. In J. Gross (Ed.). *Handbook of Emotion Regulation.* New York: Guilford Press, pp. 581-605.

Madanes, C. (1982). *Strategic Family Therapy.* Washington, DC: Jossey-Bass.

Madanes C. (1984). *Behind the One-Way Mirror: Advances in the Practice of Strategic Therapy.* San Francisco, CA: Jossey-Bass, pp. 1-30.

Marlatt, G. A. (2004). Vipassana meditation as a treatment for alcohol and drug use disorders. In S. L. Hayes, J. M. Follette, & M. M. Linehan (Eds.). *Mindfulness and Acceptance: Expanding the Cognitive-Behavioral Tradition.* New York: Guilford Press, pp. 261-287.

Meichenbaum, D. (1985). *Stress Inoculation Training.* New York: Pergamon.

Miller, A. L., Glinski, J., Woodberry, K. A., Mitchell, A. G., & Indik, J. (2002). Family therapy and dialectical behavior therapy with adolescents: Proposing a clinical synthesis. *American Journal of Psychotherapy*, 56(4), 568-584.

O'Hanlon, W. & Weiner-Davis, M. M. (1989). *In Search of Solutions: Creating a Context for Change.* New York: W. W. Norton.

Woodberry, K. A., Miller, A. L., Glinski, J., Indik, J., & Mitchell, A. G. (2002). Family therapy and dialectical behavior therapy with adolescents: A theoretical review. *The American Journal of Psychotherapy*, 56(4), 585-602.

Recommended Use of Wolpe's Subjective Units of Disturbance Scale and Quintiliani's Subjective Units of Pleasure Scale.

Simply request that the client provide a personal estimate of discomfort from 1 to 10 as a pre measure. Then provide skills or interventions; request that the client provide a post SUDS. Do the same with SUPS, which is a subjective measure of pleasure. The SUPS is used when coping and pleasure skills are the interventions. It is recommended that you use a range of 1 to 100 for both scales; this gives the client a wider range of experience to report. Changes in SUDS and SUPS over time may indicate actual changes in discomfort and pleasure.

SUDS 1 to 100: Your Score is: Pre_____Post_____

SUPS 1 to 100: Your Score is: Pre_____Post_____

8

Family Therapy for Adult Children Caregivers and Their Families

Corinne Kyriacou

*Dedicated to Jo Kay, Alan Kay, and Barbara Levine, whose immeasurable inner
strength has enabled them to effectively and lovingly take on caregiving for a
chronicall-ill parent, while maintaining peace and stability within their own families
and a presence as respected members of their professions. Their private internal
struggle is our struggle. As a society we can learn from them, but we must also do
more to ease their burden. We can start by recognizing the importance and value of
their roles in society and by better caring for their physical and emotional health.*

Abstract

Caregiving has important implications for physical health, psychological health,
and occupational and economic status (Grunfeld et al, 2004; Grant, 1999; Vitaliano,
1997). As is suggested by theorists, finding ways to better support caregivers is one
of our greatest public health challenges. Marriage and family therapists can assist
caregivers in dealing with the risks associated with caregiving. This is critical to the
quality of care provided to the care recipient, the quality of life experienced by the
caregiver, the care recipient and the extended family, as well as to the future of the
American health care system.

Introduction

Caring for aging, chronically-ill parents is becoming a way of life for
many Americans. A national caregiver survey conducted in 2004 by the
National Alliance for Caregiving and AARP found over 44 million American adults or 21 percent of the adult population, provide uncompensated
care for an adult family member or friend. The economic value of this
care has been estimated to be over $250 billion, far outstripping national
spending for nursing home care and home care combined (NAC, 2004;
Arno et al, 2002). Clearly the health care system, as well as large num-

159

bers of chronically ill Americans, is dependent upon informal caregivers. Indeed, as the population ages an increasing number of Americans will be providing care for family members and these caregivers will become an even more critical part of the health care system.

A substantial body of evidence suggests that caregiving has important implications for physical health, psychological health, and occupational and economic status (Grunfeld et al, 2004; Grant, 1999; Vitaliano, 1997). Finding ways to help caregivers deal with the risks associated with caregiving is critical to the quality of care provided to the care recipient, the quality of life experienced by the caregiver, the care recipient and the extended family, as well as to the future of the American health care system. Belle and colleagues claim that finding ways to better support caregivers is one of our greatest public health challenges (2006).

Although families have long assumed responsibility for caregiving, roles and expectations have changed dramatically as a result of the convergence of several societal changes (Levine, 2004; Lim & Zebrack, 2004; McCorkle & Pasacreta, 2001). First, advances in medical technology has enabled people to live longer with chronic illnesses, extending the period of time when family caregiving is needed. Second, sophisticated high tech home care has become more readily available enabling severely chronically-ill individuals to remain in their homes longer, but also requiring increasingly complex skills on the part of the family caregiver. Third, initiatives aimed at managing skyrocketing health care costs have shifted the burden of care from the acute care side of the health care system to the home, and consequently from formal to informal caregivers. Fourth, the number of women in the workforce has steadily increased, presenting a conflict for women who assume caregiving roles while trying to maintain professional activities and personal responsibilities associated with their immediate families. Caring for someone with a chronic illness is particularly challenging as the very definition of "chronic illness" means that the disease trajectory is unpredictable and progressive, with intensive symptom management needed to avert crises and acute episodes. Other trends, such as the aging of the population, have further changed the landscape of caregiving.

Although an increasing number of men are engaged in caregiving activities, women still represent the large majority, with an average age of forty-seven (Evercare, 2006; Donelan et al, 2002). The emotional, physical, and professional struggle of the "woman in the middle" has been eloquently charted by Elaine Brody and others (Brody, 1981, 1990; Levine, 2004). This chapter will further explore this multifaceted struggle by examining the hidden intrapersonal conflict adult daughter caregivers experience as they redefine their roles in society and their personal identities. Therapeutic techniques available to assist individuals in the transformation associated with redefining themselves to incorporate a caregiver identity will be explored using a social constructionist perspective.

Consequences of Caregiving

Numerous studies describe the impact—or burden—of caregiving on the caregiver and their families. Caregiving burden is a broad term used to describe the physical, emotional, and financial impacts of caring for someone with chronic illness (Zarit, Todd, & Zarit, 1986). Many note the presence of increased depressive symptoms, anxiety, psychosomatic symptoms, restrictions on roles and activities, strain in marital relationships, and poorer physical health among family caregivers (Evercare, 2006; Berger et al, 2005; Zarit, 2004; Levine, 2004; Faison, Faira, & Frank, 1999; Zarit et al, 1986; Sales, Schultz, & Biegel, 1990; Weitzner, Moody, & McMillan, 1997; Mor, Allen, & Siegel, 1992; Foxall & Gaston-Johansson, 1996; Wallhagen, 1992; Given et al, 1992). Level of burden has been associated with stage of care recipient's dementia, functional deficits, and behavioral disturbances. Consequences of caregiver burden are often discussed in terms of decreases in health status and quality of life. Substantial research has examined caregiver quality of life, looking at predictors that are linked to either the care recipient or the caregivers. In terms of the care recipient, age, gender, level of functioning, mental status, type of illness, and severity of pain have been found to be significantly associated with caregiver quality of life (Lim & Zebrack, 2004). In terms of caregiver characteristics, factors such as age, gender, income, initial quality of life, education, health and functional status, and mental status have been linked to quality of life (Lim & Zebrack, 2004). Additional stressors, such as caregiving demands, duration and intensity of care, problem behavior, and availability of social support have also been found to significantly impact caregiver quality of life (Lim & Zebrack, 2004).

Mockus Parks and Novielli (2000) suggest that subjective burden may be less dependent on duration of time spent caregiving, functional status, behavioral problems, and cognitive abilities of care recipient, and more so on caregiver coping and management skills. Skills associated with coping and management are typically linked to a person's level of self-efficacy and whether they have an internal or external locus of control (Lim &

Zebrack, 2004). Predisposing beliefs and attitudes toward chronic illness, locus of control, and levels of self-efficacy can all impact the ability of the adult child caregiver to adjust to their new caregiver role (Atwood & Weinstein, 2004; Bandura, 1977; Meyerowitz, 1983; Phares, 1987). Indeed, Haley et al (1987) found that coping responses were significant mediators and predictors of depression, life satisfaction, and health status. Therapeutic techniques using a social constructionist perspective can help caregivers better cope with their role change by constructing a "larger sense of the illness" and by helping the caregiver put their new role into context (Saad et al, 1995).

From a social constructionist perspective, attention should also be paid to caregiver stress associated with changes in self identity, social relationship,s and societal expectations, all of which can impact both the caregiver quality of life as well as the quality of the care they provide. Taking on substantial caregiving responsibilities for an aging parent with chronic illness can result in/require changes in an adult daughter caregiver's other roles (e.g., wife, mother, daughter, sister, friend, professional, community member). Depending on the extent of the caregiving responsibilities these "other" roles may be more or less affected. While much has been written on role strain associated with being a wife and mother while also caring for an aging parent (Levine, 2004; Faison, Faria, & Frank; 1999; Butler, Lewis, & Sunderland, 1998; Neal, 1993; Zarit, Pearlin, & Scaie, 1993), less is known about how caregiving responsibilities impact the "professional identity" and the "community member identity."

Given that the majority of caregivers are middle-aged daughters who are employed (NAC, 2004), economic impacts can be extensive. Interestingly, studies looking at economic impacts of caregiving are usually reported as lost wages, productivity costs, and absences, leaves of absences, workload reduction, or early retirement (MetLife, 2006). Less attention is given to caregiver stress associated with trying to maintain a professional identity while managing complicated caregiving tasks, or for those who ultimately give up the fight of balancing work and caregiving, the subsequent loss of professional identity. The loss of this aspect of self can be particularly stressful for middle-aged adult women who may have just recently entered a phase in their lives when they are able to dedicate themselves to their careers after many years of childrearing-related obligations, or who may have just recently reached a level within their careers that took years to achieve. The resulting intrapersonal conflict can put the adult daughter at risk for an identity crisis, particularly if the role of caregiver is perceived by the caregiver as less valued by their professional community, or society at large, than their previous role as professional, productive, economic contributor. Definitions of occupational burden need to include stress associated with identity conflict. Reconciling desire to "do what's right" for elderly parents versus to "do what's good" for adult daughter caregivers can cause cognitive conflicts, which can lead to emotional distress.

The socially-constructed "caregiver self" can incorporate positive elements from the previous self-identity, or it can overwhelm the previous self-identity putting the caregiver at great risk for psychological and physiological crisis. How the caregiver experiences their role transformation, how well they accept and manage the integration of their past self and their new self, and how they perceive their social world to experience their new role, will determine the caregiver self-identity and the ability of the caregiver to provide quality care while maintaining a high quality life of their own.

Common Interventions for Caregivers

The National Family Caregiver Support Program (NFCSP), established by the Older Americans Act Amendment of 2000, Title III-E, urges the aging network to treat caregivers as direct consumers with needs distinct from care recipients. Given the wide range of challenges associated with caring for the chronically ill, numerous interventions have been developed. NFCSP identifies five service areas of caregiving interventions and resources: 1) Information; 2) Assistance; 3) Counseling; 4) Respite; and, 5) Supplemental services. The availability and effectiveness of common interventions focused on these areas are briefly reviewed here.

Information, assistance, and referral services have long been considered the most needed caregiver services (Friss, 1990). Regardless of how highly functioning the caregiver, care recipient, and extended family relationships are, caregivers always need help with accessing relevant and current information and with finding helpful assistance, appropriate referrals, and high quality services. However, much has been written on the fact that in and of itself, information not a sufficient intervention (Kennet et al, 2000). Additionally, caregiver and family needs typically vary across the course of a disease as well as in response to life changes external to the caregiving relationship. Information and services useful at one point may not be helpful at another, suggesting that periodic or ongoing assistance is often warranted (Whittier, Coon, & Aaker, 2001;

Levine, 2004). Furthermore, even when services are available, many caregivers remain unaware of them (Maslow & Selstad, 2001).

Outcomes differ depending on what type of information was provided and how it was provided. Informational interventions involving the distribution of written brochures or phone numbers may have poorer outcomes than interventions involving a support group, hands-on workshop, or where an actual linkage to the needed service is facilitated (Weuve, Boult, & Morishita, 2000; Cole, Griffin, & Ruiz, 1986). On the other hand, not all caregivers feel comfortable with the support group/workshop approach and need to be able to access information in other, less direct ways (Schmall, 1995; Levine, 2004). The effectiveness of the intervention, particularly when dealing with information, education, and referral services, depends on the availability, accessibility, appropriateness, acceptability, and affordability of services.

The category labeled Counseling includes individual counseling, organization of support groups, and caregiver training to assist caregivers in making decisions and solving problems relating to their caregiving roles. Support groups are by far the most common type of counseling intervention and they exist in various forms: online groups, telephone groups, hospital-based groups, nursing home-based groups, community-based or social service agency groups, or groups affiliated with religious organizations. Support groups are generally designed to provide informal peer support, information about diseases and disability, and referrals for caregiver support services. Studies have shown that participants in support groups typically evaluate these programs as quite useful and helpful (Levine, 2004; Butler, Lewis, & Sunderland, 1998; Whittier, Coon, & Aaker, 2001; Gonyea, 1989; Toseland, Rossiter, & Labrecque, 1989). In addition, there is some evidence that they provide knowledge and enhance informal support networks (Bourgeois, Schultz, & Burgio, 1996). However, there is much less evidence of their effectiveness in improving caregiver mental and physical health or ability to manage their caregiving responsibilities (Levine, 2004; Dura, Stukenberg, & Kiecolt-Glaser, 1991; Monahan, Greene, & Coleman, 1992; Russo, Vitaliano, & Brewer, 1995). While a considerable number of studies have examined the effectiveness of psychosocial interventions for caregiver and family distress, findings vary with regards to individual versus group interventions (Knight et al, 1993; Klausner & Alexopolos, 1999).

Whittier, Coon, & Aaker (2001) reviewed available studies of caregiver interventions, and found greater improvements in outcomes to be associated with more comprehensive interventions. Programs that combine a number of necessary components such as support services, skills training, counseling, and education have been found to be particularly promising (Kennett et al, 2000; Zarit; 2004; Levine, 2004; Kosloski & Montgomery, 1993; Mittleman et al, 1996; Mohide et al, 1990; Montgomery & Borgatta, 1989; Ostwald, Hepburn, Caron, Burns, & Mantell , 1999; Seltzer, Ivry, & Litchfield, 1987; Zarit et al, 1998). Members of Kaiser Permanente-Northeast, a regional HMO, participated in a study comparing the Health Education Group Intervention (HEP), a multi-component program, and the staff model of "usual care" offered to caregivers. Participants in the HEP group were found to have lower rates of depression, greater social integration, increased effectiveness in solving pressing problems, increased knowledge of community services and how to access them, improved feelings of competence, and enhanced responses to the caregiving situation (Toseland, Smith, & McCallion, 2001). However, no association was found between the HEP intervention and improvements in caregiver burden, role strain, or the physical and emotional demands of caregiving. Others have found that multi-component psycho-educational interventions can significantly reduce caregivers' negative reactions to disruptive behaviors and caregiver burden over time (Ostwald et al, 1999) and even substantially increase the time caregivers are able to care for patients at home (Mittleman et al, 1996). A major challenge associated with multi-component programs is the difficulty in teasing out which specific interventions are most helpful, limiting the development of targeted, cost-effective treatments for caregivers (Whittier et al, 2001).

The counseling category also includes traditional psychotherapy, individual problem-solving, and couples, group, and family therapy. A range of psychotherapeutic techniques have been used to relieve caregiver depression and anxiety, resolve pre-existing personal problems, which can complicate caregiving, reconcile conflicts between the caregivers and recipient, and/or improve family functioning (Levine, 2004; Whittier et al, 2001; Butler, Lewis & Sunderland, 1998). Some data suggest that greater improvements in emotional health are found for daughters and daughters-in-law of frail elderly parents when receiving individual counseling (Toseland, Rossiter, Peak, & Smith, 1990). However others report that greater gains can be found when the caregiver-care recipient is counseled as a structural unit, incorporating the family of the caregiver (Atwood & Weinstein, 2004; Butler, Lewis, & Sunderland, 1998). Increasingly common is a combination of individual and family therapy for caregivers and their families. Atwood and Weinstein (2004) state that when one member of a family is faced with a serious illness, the emotional well-being of the entire family system is threatened.

The effectiveness of family counseling for caregivers and care recipients varies across ethnic groups. Belle and colleagues (2006) evaluated Cuban American and Caucasian caregivers in Miami who were exposed to the Family-Based Structural Multisystem In-Home Intervention, which provides family counseling to identify existing communication problems and to produce changes in interaction patterns so that caregivers are better able to solicit available family and community resources. The focus of change is on the interaction between the individual and the environment, an interaction that is considered to be embedded within larger social and cultural systems (Coon, Schultz, & Ory, 1999). Positive mental health outcomes have been found with this intervention, particularly for Cuban-American caregivers (Czaja & Rubert, 2002).

Caregivers with high levels of emotional distress have been found to benefit from psychotherapy grounded in a number of theoretical orientations, including cognitive behavioral therapy, psychodynamic therapy, intergenerational family therapy, and others (Atwood & Weinstein, 2004; Whittier et al, 2001; Butler, Lewis, & Sunderland, 1998; Gallagher-Thompson and Steffen, 1994). Various approaches have been found to be moderately successful at helping caregivers with emotional distress associated with role conflict (e.g., mother-daughter; husband-wife; mother-children), role strain and burden, and subsequent depression and anxiety; however, few have honed in on the potentially powerful influence of an internal identity crisis on the part of the caregiver resulting from the social construction of a caregiver identity.

The Social Construction of the Caregiver Self

Conflicts associated with role change, resulting lifestyle interference, and relationship adjustment, have been the focus of a growing number of studies (National Family Caregiver Association & National Alliance for Caregiving, 2002; Jones & Peters, 1992; Boyle et al, 2000; Cameron, Franche, Cheung, & Stewart, 2002; Nijboer, Treimstar, Tempelaar, Sanderman, & Van den bos, 1999; Dunn, Bonner, Lewis, & Meize-Grochowski, 1994). Yet, more often than not, role change is narrowly defined as the addition of new tasks or needing to make adjustments to relationships. Alternatively, role change can be more broadly defined, recognizing the process of change, and the need for a new social construction of identity to occur.

Women take on new roles several times throughout their lives; becoming a wife and a mother are two of the most complex transformations in terms of modified identity. However, in both of these cases, and also when they become a professional, society views the transformation as an achievement, as an exciting, life-enriching progressive change in identity. The social construction of the wife-self and mother-self is based on new membership within a vibrant community of mothers and wives. On the other hand, the transformation from a daughter to a caregiving daughter is typically met with far less enthusiasm. Indeed, the transformation begins with recognition that a loved one's health is in decline. The social construction of caring for someone with a chronic illness "involves a construction of a reality centered around the concepts of sickness and disease, often involving isolation and control" (Atwood & Weinstein, 2004). While there may be many other caregivers with whom the new caregiver can share experiences and derive support from, these others are usually dispersed and hidden. Outside of support groups, caregivers do not represent a cohesive community whose membership is perceived as an achievement or life goal.

The change associated with the caregiver's "role" starts at the time of diagnosis, goes through many iterations during the course of the illness and as a result of other life changes, and continues long after the caregiving has ended. Furthermore, there is not just one role that needs to change for caregiving to be a manageable and rewarding experience; caregivers need to successfully transform multiple roles and the ability to do this is largely dependent on their socially-constructed concept of self. The case study example below presents one example of how becoming a caregiver can affect multiple roles and relationships and how these changes can impact a caregiver's personal and social identity.

Case Study Example

An adult daughter used to shop, have lunch and confide in her elderly but highly functioning mother about work, marriage, parenting, even politics. Frequent conversations took place over the phone and in person. Then, one day the elderly mother experienced a massive stroke and is rendered unable to speak or perform any activities of daily living or instrumental activities on her own. Furthermore, the elderly mother's cognitive abilities are greatly compromised. In addition to the new and often unpleasant tasks associated with the actual caregiving, the adult daughter is no longer able to communicate with her mother over the phone and only in a very limited way in person. The adult daughter has lost her best friend and confidant. Numerous administrative tasks have added considerable time burden to the daughter's already busy schedule. Her husband and children are sympathetic, but they also need their wife/mother to fulfill her established roles in their lives, which becomes increasingly difficult. Her friends are concerned but also frustrated with her gloominess and distraction. The adult daughter's workplace is generous with time-off in the beginning, but quickly loses patience with her lack of focus and drive. She loses a coveted promotion after cancelling several business trips and presentations to remain at home with her mother. Juggling direct caregiving, home care scheduling, health care appointments and the associated paperwork becomes too much for the working caregiver who first attempts part-time and then ultimately resigns from her professional position. Society used to see an enviable relationship between a successful, professional adult daughter and a regal-looking elderly mother who would walk arm in arm, chatting and laughing. Now they see a grief-stricken, stressed out woman wheeling her disabled elderly mother, in silence. Whereas before the duo was vibrant and dynamic and full-fledged members of the social fabric that makes up society, now the duo is viewed as representing filial obligation, regret, burden, and sympathy.

Gender identity is a dominant component of self that affects values, attitudes, and behavior (Kramer, 2005). Female caregivers more so than male caregivers, tend to forgo institutionalization of care recipients even when care demands are overwhelming. Stereotypical female gender traits that support and facilitate the enduring of burden are often intertwined in a woman's definitions of self (Kramer, 2005). Carol Levine (2004) discusses how caregiving has historically been perceived as "women's work" and that this societal expectation persists despite dramatic advances in equality. So entrenched in the female make-up is this expectation that thinking or acting outside its traditional parameters is cause for great internal strife.

Joel Best states that "social problems are what people view as social problems, and no condition is a social problem until someone considers it to be" (Best, 1995). Is caregiving a social problem? Is it related to the undervaluing of women's work in general? Is it an outcome of ageism or disdain for the sick? Are caregivers seen as lesser citizens because their work is seen as having little economic value? Interestingly, despite the substantial numbers of Americans who are providing care for elderly parents, caregiving relationships and activities are typically unseen and unheard. While there has certainly been an increase in awareness of and research on caregiving issues, dialogue and discourse about caregiving remain largely within specific academic and policy circles or within the private family unit.

Great improvements have been made in the availability and range of interventions available to assist caregivers; however many caregivers still perceive their membership in society to be on the fringe. Many feel disconnected from the mainstream as they watch the strong, independent, free majority lead productive lives, while they feel devalued by society, ignored and desperate. Carol Levine (2004) asserts that despite the fact that caregiving is not an isolated issue, most caregivers feel isolated, cut off from the rest of society. Caregivers may not see themselves as a member of any group; they need help in reconstructing that view to one that identifies them as members of a growing, helping army of adults juggling caregiving with other life activities.

Caregiving can be thought of as representing familial loyalty and devotion, as adhering to traditional family values, as daughters fulfilling roles expected of them. Alternatively, caregiving can be thought of as representing sacrifice, burden, obligation and failure on the part of the health or social service system. Caregivers will redefine their identities based on how they think society views the activities and tasks associated with caregiving. They can either see themselves as contributing members of a productive society, fulfilling a valued, respected, needed role in society, or they can see themselves as locked into a caregiving relationship that is pitied, ignored, misunderstood, and outside the mainstream. Believing that the role they play in society is commonly understood, respected, and valued will help caregivers make a healthy transformation to a caregiver self.

The construction of the caregiver self is likely dependent on how the caregiver thinks they are defined by both their family and by society. If the care recipient can define boundaries, show gratitude, and honor the rights of the caregiver, then the caregiver can more readily accept the new identity and integrate it into their existing identity. If the caregiver's children can show interest in and patience with the caregiving relationship, the caregiver can more readily accept the new identity and integrate it into their existing identity. If the caregiver's spouse can show compassion and understanding for the caregiving relationship, the caregiver can more readily accept the new identity and integrate in into their existing identity. If the caregiver's professional community can show flexibility and commitment to helping the caregiver balance their work and caring responsibilities, the caregiver can more readily accept the new identity and integrate it into their existing identity. If the physician community can treat caregivers as valued members of the care team—both through active solicitation of information and by imparting critical information—then the caregiver can more readily accept the new identity and integrate it into their existing identity. Finally, if the larger social community—through caregiver-friendly policies and programs and open, candid dialogue—can show respect for and attribute value to the caregiving relationship, the caregiver can more readily accept the new identity and integrate it into their existing identity.

In reality, it is unlikely that all these potential scenarios will converge to establish the kind of supportive structure caregivers would need to make and sustain an emotionally sound transformation to caregiver. Children, spouses, chronically-ill parents, providers, employers, policymakers, and other community stakeholders are struggling with their own competing interests and demands, and in many cases are unable to demonstrate the kind of empathy and supports needed. Family therapy can help the caregiver redefine their identity within the context of the real world, while simultaneously guiding those who are most influential in the social construction of the caregiver self to change their behavior, minimizing destructive social influences.

The Potential of Therapeutic Techniques Grounded in Social Constructionist Theory

The structural approach to family therapy defines the family as a unit undergoing constant transformation, and assumes that many problems within the unit stem from harmful, external social forces. By focusing on the social construction of such realities—in the case of caregiving perhaps lesser citizenship, prejudice against the sick, ageism, economic oppression—the structural approach takes the focus off the individual exclusively and emphasizes the interaction between the individual and their social environment. The structural approach to family therapy was originally developed by Salvador Minuchin (1999) who defined the therapist's role as an active, intervening one where the family reality is challenged and reconstructed to promote enhanced functioning. Key to social constructionist therapy is the co-creation by therapists and clients of new, more satisfying and positive "stories" or "scripts" (Atwood & Weinstein, 2004) that have the potential to help caregivers better cope with their transforming self and accept their new identity.

Emotional distress is not always readily apparent. A caregiver may be going through the motions, keeping it all together on the outside, when on the inside there is hidden intrapersonal conflict. They may understand the parameters of their new role quite well, efficiently and effectively progressing through the various stages associated with caregiving. However, what they are saying to themselves, how they are interpreting their place in the world, how they think their children, family, and social world perceive them may be significantly different from what would be expected given their day-to-day appearance and behavior. Social constructionist therapists will attempt to uncover the existing definitions of self and help caregivers reconcile disparate thought processes while reconstructing realities that can bring inner peace.

Caregivers need a safe forum to express their deeply hidden thoughts and concerns, which define their identities. They need to be able to reconcile the seemingly contradictory thoughts of "I am giving back to my mother who raised me" with "I am sacrificing the prime of my life," which left to simmer can breed dangerous internal conflict and emotional distress. Caregivers need language to express the discomfort associated with parent-child role reversal, which can lead to intense sadness and anxiety, particularly in the face of simultaneous parenting and caregiving. Shamed and angered by their feelings of exasperation and inadequacies can lead to further retreat and separation from family, friends, colleagues, and community. Increased stress and isolation can lead to decreases in physical and emotional health, both of which will negatively impact quality of life and quality of care for both the caregiver and the care recipient.

Caregivers need to be taught to reconstruct their caregiving role in positive ways: as representing opportunities for modeling behavior for their own children; spending quality time with their parent; giving back to the community; and helping to build an infrastructure that enables the health care system to function. They need to learn how to share responsibilities without feeling guilty, to vent or cry about their struggle or ask for help without feeling like a failure or bad daughter. They need to learn how to incorporate the caregiver role into their identity without letting it define them. They need to learn how to command respect from the health care system of which they are vital members. They need help finding ways to balance new constraints with satisfying professional and personal outlets.

Tronto (1993) distinguishes among four components that make up caring relationships. They include general "caring about" activities such as remembering someone with a phonecall; "taking care of" activities such as coordination and oversight of services; "direct caring" activities, which include the physical labor associated with caregiving; and "receiving care," which takes into consideration the reciprocal nature of caring. Bella (2006) claims that women tend to enmesh these four components, making assumptions that "good caregiving" must incorporate all four aspects. If the adult daughter either cannot provide the direct care or agonizes over it because of competing obligations or expectations, feelings of guilt and failure may arise. Social constructionist therapy can help caregivers differentiate among the various components of caring by rewriting internal scripts or beliefs about what represents "good enough" care.

Families, too, need guidance with communication, conflict resolution, and reconstructing the meaning of illness, caregiving, and family.

Predisposing beliefs and attitudes towards chronic illness and ability to control outcomes may differ greatly across family members causing confusion and stress on the family system. This could be particularly threatening to the caregiver-care recipient relationship. The care recipient may become more isolated and dependent as the caregiver takes on more controlling attributes, creating a vicious cycle of anger and resentment, guilt and sadness. The quality of the pre-illness relationship and how the caregiver perceives their role and status in the family and within society will greatly impact how the new reality is socially constructed by the caregiver and their family members. It is this social context that dictates both intra- and interpersonal scripts for behavior—that is, self talk and conversation within the caregiver and between the caregiver, care recipient, the caregiver's family, and members of the community (Atwood & Weinstein, 2004). Therapy can help caregivers and their families establish, negotiate, rewrite, and/or redefine scripts so that roles are mutually understood and accepted, and so that communication and subsequent satisfaction with relationships can be improved. Family therapists using a social constructionist approach can assist the family in saying goodbye to their pre-illness expectations, and help them accept and adjust to their new reality by establishing boundaries for the illness and limiting its defining power (Schultz, 2000; Atwood & Weinstein, 2004). Without appropriate limits, the change associated with illness and caregiving can be overwhelming for a family, threatening their ability to function as individuals and as a familial unit.

Implications for Family Therapy and Family Medicine

A 2006 Evercare Survey of over 500 caregivers found stress to be the second most common health problem for caregivers (70%), preceded by energy and sleep (87%), and followed by pain (60%) and depression (52%). Although the need for intervention is serious and extensive, a number of obstacles to getting needed care persist.

First, little attention is paid to the mental health or the status of the family during a physician office visit. While the majority of caregivers report that their doctor or their care recipient's doctor is aware of their caregiving role, only 56 percent say they have ever had discussions with these physicians about how to improve their health (Evercare, 2006). Restrictions on time coupled with a continued focus on the medical model as opposed to the biopsychosocial model, has resulted in fewer referrals to mental health services. Atwood & Weinstein (2004) urge medical practitioners to expand their perspective from an exclusive focus on the individual patient to a social systemic model focusing on the family (Atwood & Weinstein, 2004).

Furthermore, addressing caregiver or family stress may be perceived by the physician as "outside the scope" of her responsibility. However, because caregiving has been found to be associated with decreases in health for the caregiver, as well as decreased quality of care provided by the caregiver, consequences of stress associated with caregiving—whether a result of time constraints, identity conflict, or any other reason—is a problem the family physicians must address. Physicians need to be more aware of the range of negative emotional and physical outcomes that can result in excess morbidity and mortality.

Second, while the trend may be changing, primary care physicians remain largely unaware of the range of screening tools and the types of therapeutic interventions available for referral. There are a number of excellent office-based risk screens available for physician use, and enhanced medical training in conjunction with improved partnerships between family medicine and family therapy can raise physician awareness.

Third, Heru and Ryan (2002) found that although caregivers report depressive symptoms and family dysfunction, they often refuse suggested treatment, stating that their problems are situational, that they do not have the time for treatment or because they are conflicted about the meaning of and purpose of caregiver interventions. Caregivers may have a socially-constructed perception about what the health care system thinks of "the need" for treatment. They may believe that physicians and others think therapeutic interventions are only needed for weak caregivers. They may feel guilt, shame, or anger at the suggestion of mental health intervention.

Family physicians need to incorporate techniques from the social constructionist perspective to help caregivers revise this dangerous belief. In addition, changes in physician behavior towards caregivers can go far in helping caregivers define their caregiving role and status in the health system and society at large. If primary care physicians treated caregivers as partners, if they drew upon information and advice offered by caregivers instead of just being directive, this would change the social construction of the caregiver identity.

Fourth, Butler, Lewis, and Sunderland (1998) explain that it is not uncommon for an older person to be brought into a therapists' office by an adult child caregiver, when in actuality it is the adult caregiver who needs the help, or even more likely the family that needs help dealing with changes to the system. Family therapists must be on alert for caregivers at risk presenting themselves in various ways.

There are many other factors that have the potential to impact whether and how caregivers interact with the health care system that need to be further explored. How culture and ethnicity mediate the caregiver experience, their presentation of distress and the response of the medical field, needs to be examined. Assumptions about attitudes towards caregiving across different ethnic groups need to be addressed by both family physicians and family therapists. Whether and how the care recipient's diagnosis and level of disease severity impact caregiver interpretations of their role is important to understand. How the hypothesized socially-constructed caregiver self differs for adult male children caregivers or spouses-as-caregivers or parents-as-caregivers should also be further examined. What therapeutic technique yields greatest benefit for caregivers and their families is yet unknown. Rigorous program evaluation is essential for the development of high quality, effective caregiver interventions. Targeted and realistic outcome measures are needed to ensure caregiver interventions are evidence-based (Schulz, 2000; Bourgeiois et al, 1996). Finally, issues related to cost, access, and availability of psychotherapeutic interventions using a social constructionist perspective needs to be explored.

Family physicians serve as the gateway to care for caregivers. They are in a particularly critical position to assist caregivers by screening for stress to prevent physical burnout and illness or emotional crisis (Levine, 2004; Mockus Parks & Novielli, 2000). They must do a better job at getting caregivers at risk into treatment. Family physicians need to consider the origins of the stress and resulting complaints, and incorporate referrals to family therapy into their usual care.

References

Arno, P.S. (2002). *Economic Value of Informal Caregiving*. Orlando, FL: Annual Meeting of the American Association of Geriatric Psychiatry.

Atwood, J. & Weinstein, E. (2004). Family practice, family therapy: A collaboration of dialogue. *Psychology Online*. Retrieved November 21, 2007 from *www.priory.com*.

Bandura, A. (1977). Self-efficacy: Toward a unifying theory of behavioral change. *Psychological Review*, 84, 191-215.

Belle, S.H., Burgio, L., Burns, R., Coon, D., Czaja, S.J., Gallagher-Thompson et al (2006). Enhancing the quality of life of dementia caregivers from different ethnic or racial groups: A randomized, controlled trial. *Annals of Internal Medicine*, 145(10), 727-38.

Berger, G., Bernhardt, T., Weimer, E., Peters, J., Kratzsch, T., & Frolich, L. (2005). Longitudinal study on the relationship between symptomatology of dementia and levels of subjective burden and depression among family caregivers in memory clinic patients. *Journal of Geriatric Psychiatry and Neurology*, 18(3), 119-128.

Best, J. (1995). *Images of Issues: Typifying Contemporary Social Problems*. New York: Aldine De Gruyter.

Bourgeois, M., Schulz, R., & Burgio, L. (1996). Interventions for caregivers of patients with Alzheimer's disease: A review and analysis of content, process, and outcomes. *International Journal on Aging and Human Development*, 43, 35-92.

Brody, E. (1981). "Women in the middle" and family help to older people. *The Gerontologist*, 21(5), 471-80.

Brody, E. M. (1990). Women, work, and parent care. *Women in the Middle: Their Parent Care Years* (pp. 213-229). New York: Springer Publishing.

Boyle, D. et al (2000). Caregiver quality of life after autologous bone marrow transplantation. *Cancer Nursing*, 23, 193-203.

Butler, R. N., Lewis, M. I., & Sunderland, T. (1998). *Aging and Mental Health*, 5th Edition. Boston, MA: Allyn and Bacon.

Cameron, J. I., Franche, R., Cheung, A. M., & Stewart, D. E. (2002). Lifestyle interference and emotional distress in family caregivers of advanced cancer patients. *Cancer*, 94, 521-527.

Cole, L., Griffin, K, & Ruiz, B. (1986). A comprehensive approach to working with families of Alzheimer's patients. In R. Dobrof (Ed.), *Social Work and Alzheimer's Disease (pp. 27-39).* New York: Haworth.

Coon, D., Schulz, R., & Ory, M. (1999). Innovative intervention approaches with Alzheimer's disease caregivers. In D. Biegel & A. Blum (Eds.), *Innovations in Practice and Service Delivery across the Lifespan* (pp. 295-325). New York: Oxford University Press.

Czaja, S. J., & Rubert, M. P. (2002). Telecommunications technology as an aid to family caregivers of persons with dementia. *Psychosomatic Medicine*, 64(3):469-76.

Donelan, K., et al (2002). Challenged to care: Informal caregivers in a changing health care system. *Health Affairs*, July/August, 222-231.

Dunn, S. A., Bonner, P. N., Lewis, S. L., & Meize-Grochowsku, R. (1994). Quality of life for spouses of CAPD patients. *American Nephrology Nurses Association Journal*, 21, 237-247.

Dura, J., Stukenberg, K., & Kiecolt-Glaser, J. (1991). Anxiety and depressive disorders in adult children caring for demented parents. *Psychology and Aging*, 6, 467-473.

Evercare & National Alliance for Caregiving. (2006). *Evercare Study of Caregivers in Decline: A Close up Look at the Health Risks of Caring for a Loved One. Report of Findings.* Minnetonka, MN: Author as Publisher.

Faison, K. J., Faria, S. H., & Frank, D. (1999). Caregivers of chronically ill elderly: Perceived burden. *Journal of Community Health*, 16(4), 243-53.

Foxall, M. J. & Gaston-Johansson, F. (1996). Burden and health outcomes of family caregivers of hospitalized bone marrow transplant patients. *Journal of Advanced Nursing*, 24(5), 915-23.

Friss, L. (1990). A model state-level approach to family survival for caregivers of brain-impaired adults. *The Gerontologist*, 30, 121-125.

Gallagher-Thompson, D., & Steffen, A. (1994). Comparative effects of cognitive-behavioral and brief psychodynamic psychotherapies for depressed family caregivers. *Journal of Consulting and Clinical Psychology*, 62, 543-549.

Given, C., Given, B., Stommel, M., Collins, C., King, S., & Franklin, S. (1992). The caregiver reaction assessment (CRA) for caregivers to persons with chronic physical and mental impairments. *Research in Nursing and Health*, 15, 271–283.

Gonyea, J. (1989). Alzheimer's disease support groups: An analysis of their structure, format and perceived benefits. *Social Work in Health Care*, 14(1), 61-72.

Grant, I. (1999). Caregiving may be hazardous to your health. *Psychosomatic Medicine*, 61, 420-423.

Grunfeld, E., Coyle, D., Whelan, T., Clinch, J., Reyno, L., Earle, C. C., Wilan, A., Viola, R., Coristine, M., Janz, T., and Glossop, R. (2004). Family caregiver burden: Results of a longitudinal study of breast cancer patients and their principal caregivers. *Canadian Medical Association Journal*, 170(12), 1795-801.

Haley, W. E., Brown, S. L., & Levine, E. G. (1987). Experimental evaluation of the effectiveness of group intervention for dementia caregivers. *The Gerontologist*, 27, 377-383.

Heru, A.M. & Ryan, C.E. (2002). Depressive symptoms and family functioning in the caregivers of recently hospitalized patients with chronic/recurrent mood disorders. *International Journal of Psychosocial Rehabilitation*, 7, 53-60.

Jones, D. A. S., & Peters, T. J. (1992). Caring for elderly dependents: Effects on the carer's quality of life. *Age and Ageing*, 21, 421-428.

Kennet, J., Burgio, L., & Schulz, R. (2000). Interventions for in-home caregivers: A review of research 1990 to present. In R. Schulz (Ed.), *Handbook of Dementia Caregiving* (pp. 61-125). New York: Springer.

Klausner, E. J., & Alexopoulos, G. S. (1999). The Future of Psychosocial Treatments for Elderly Patients. *Psychiatric Services*, 50(9), 1198-1204.

Kosloski, K., & Montgomery, R. (1993). Perceptions of respite services as predictors of utilization. *Research on Aging*, 15, 399 - 314.

Kramer, M. K. (2005). Self-characterization of adult female informal caregivers: Gender identity and the bearing of burden. *Research and Theory in Nursing Practice*, 19(2), 137-61.

Knight, B. G., Lutsky, S. M., & Macofsky-Urban, F. (1993). A meta-analytic review of interventions for caregiver distress: Recommendations for future research. *Gerontologist*, 33, 240-248.

Levine, C. (Ed.) (2004). Always *on Call: When Illness Turns Families into Caregivers*. A United Hospital Fund Book. Nashville, TN: Vanderbilt University Press.

Lim, J. & Zebrack, B. (2004). Caring for family members with chronic physical illness: A critical review of caregiver literature. *Health and Quality of Life Outcomes*, 2, 50-59.

Maslow, K., & Selstad, J. (2001). Chronic Care Networks for Alzheimer's disease: Approaches for involving and supporting family caregivers in an innovative model of dementia care. *Alzheimer's Care Quarterly*, 2, 33-46.

McCorkle, R., & Pasacreta, J. V. (2001). Enhancing Caregiver Outcomes in Palliative Care. *Cancer Control*, 8(1), 36-45.

MetLife and the National Alliance for Caregiving. (2006). *The MetLife Caregiving Cost Study: Productivity Losses to U.S. Businesses*. Westport, CT: Publisher as Author.

Meyerowitz, B. E. (1983). Postmastectomy coping strategies and the quality of life. *Health Psychology*, 2, 117-132.

Minuchin, S. (1999). Retelling, reimagining and re-searching: A continuing conversation. *Journal of Marriage and Family Therapy*, 25(1), 9-14.

Mittelman, M., Ferris, S., Shulman, E., Steinberg, G., & Levin, B. (1996) Family intervention to delay nursing home placement of patients with Alzheimer's disease. *Journal of the American Medical Association*, 276, 1725-1731.

Mockus Parks, S. & Novielli, K. D. (2000). A Practical Guide to Caring for Caregivers. *American Family Physician*, 62, 2613-20; 2621-2.

Mohide, E., Pringle, D., Streiner, D., Gilbert, J., Muir, G., & Tew, M. (1990). A randomized trial of family caregiver support in the home management of dementia. *Journal of the American Geriatrics Society*, 38, 446-454.

Monahan, D., Greene, V., & Coleman, P. (1992). Caregiver support groups: Factors affecting service use. *Social Work*, 37, 254-260.

Montgomery, R., & Borgatta, E. (1989). The effects of alternative support strategies on family caregiving. *The Gerontologist*, 29, 457-464.

Mor, V., Allen, S. M., Siegel, K., & Houts, P. (1992). Determinants of need and unmet need among cancer patients residing at home. *Health Services Research*, 27(3), 337-60.

National Alliance for Caregiving & AARP. (1997). *Family Caregiving in the U.S.: Findings from a National Survey.* Washington, DC.

National Family Caregiver Association & National Alliance for Caregiving (2002). *Self-Awareness in Family Caregiving: A Report on the Communications Environment.* Kensington, MD: Author as Publisher.

Neal, M. (1993). *Balancing Work, and Caregiving for Children, Adults and Elders.* Thousand Oaks, CA: Sage Publications.

Nijboer, C., Triemstar, M., Tempelaar, R., Sanderman, R., & Van den bos, G. A. M. (1999). Determinants of caregiving experiences and mental health of partners of cancer patients. *Cancer*, 86, 577-588.

Ostwald, S., Hepburn, K., Caron, W., Burns, T., & Mantell, R. (1999). Reducing caregiver burden: A randomized psychoeducational intervention for caregivers of persons with dementia. *The Gerontologist*, 39, 299-309.

Phares, E. J. (1987). Locus of control. In R. J. Corsini (Eds.). *Concise Encyclopedia of Psychology.* New York: Wiley.

Russo, J., Vitaliano, P. P., Brewer, D. D., Katon, W., & Becker, J. (1995). Psychiatric disorders in spouse caregivers of care recipients with Alzheimer's disease and matched controls: a diathesis-stress model of psychopathology. *Journal of Abnormal Psychology*, 104(1), 197-204.

Saad, K., Hartman, J., Ballard, C., Kurian, M., Graham, C., and Wilcock, G. (1995). Coping by the carers of dementia sufferers. *Age and Ageing*, 24, 495-498.

Sales, E., Schultz, R., & Biegel, D. (1990). Predictors of strain in families of cancer patients: a review of the literature. *Journal of Psychosocial Oncology*, 10, 1-26.

Schmall, V. L. (1995). Family caregiver education and training: Enhancing self-efficacy. *Journal of Case Management*, 4(4), 156-62.

Schulz, R. (2000). *Handbook of Dementia Caregiving.* New York: Springer.

Seltzer, M., Ivry, J., & Litchfield, L. (1987). Family members as case managers: Partnership between the formal and informal support networks. *The Gerontologist*, 27, 722-728.

Toseland, R., Rossiter, C., & Labrecque, M. (1989). The effectiveness of peer led and professionally led groups to support family caregivers. *The Gerontologist*, 29, 465-471.

Toseland, R., Rossiter, C., Peak, T., & Smith, G. (1990). Comparative effectiveness of individual and group interventions to support family caregivers. *Social Work*, 35, 209-217.

Toseland, R., Smith, G., & McCallion, P. (2001). Family caregivers of the frail elderly. In A. Gutterman (Ed.), *Handbook of Social Work Practice with Vulnerable and Resilient Populations* (pp. 548-581). New York: Columbia University Press.

Tronto, J. (1993). *Moral Boundaries: A Political Argument for an Ethic of Care.* New York: Routledge.

Vitaliano, P. P. (1997). Physiological and physical concomitants to caregiving: Introduction to a special issue. *Annals of Behavior and Medicine*, 19, 75-77.

Wallhagen, M. I. (1992). Caregiving demands: Their difficulty and effects on the well-being of elderly caregivers. *Scholarly Inquiry Nursing Practice*, 6 (2), 111-133.

Weitzner, M., Moody, L., & McMillan, S. (1997). Symptom management issues in hospice care. *American Journal of Hospital Palliative Care.* 14(4), 190–195.

Weuve, J., Boult, C., & Morishita, L. (2000). The effects of outpatient geriatric evaluation and management on caregiver burden. *The Gerontologist*, 40, 429-436.

Whittier, S., Coon, D., & Aaker, J. (2001). Caregiver Support Interventions. In *Family Caregivers in California: Needs, Interventions and Model Programs.* Berkeley,

CA: University of California at Berkeley, Center for Advanced Studies of Aging Services.

Zarit, S. H. (2004). Family care and burden at the end of life. *Canadian Medical Association Journal*, 170(12), 1811-2.

Zarit, S. H., Pearlin, L. I., & Warner Schaie, K. (1993). *Caregiving Systems: Formal and Informal Helpers*. Mahwah, NJ: Lawrence Erlbaum Associates, Inc.

Zarit, S., Stephens, M., Townsend, A., & Greene, R. (1998). Stress reduction for family caregivers: Effects of adult day care use. *Journal of Gerontology: Social Sciences,* 53B, S267-S277.

Zarit, S.H., Todd, P.A., & Zarit, J.M. (1986). Subjective burden of husbands and wives as caregivers: A longitudinal study. *The Gerontologist*, 26(3), 260-266.

9

The Chronically Ill and End-of-Life Care

Jayne Gassman

Abstract

This chapter explores the concept of a good death. To determine the good death, researchers investigated how people want to be cared for at the end of their lives. They identified five goals for quality end-of-life care. They are to (1) avoid inappropriately prolonged dying, (2) to strengthen relationships with loved ones, (3) to relieve the burden on their loved ones and (4) to receive adequate pain and symptom management. Family therapists can assist their clients by educating families with a dying member concerning these wishes.

Billy was actively dying of AIDs. The day he died, his family was at his side. Before AIDs-related dementia ravaged his mind, pop music had been a great joy in his life, so his family played his favorite songs over and over again. They told family stories. They laughed and cried. They touched and stroked his face. When his pillow was damp they turned it over. They held his hands and said their final goodbyes as he departed this life for the next. His sister said,

> The bed creaked when he died. You could hear his body settle into the bed...but, maybe, he was just getting up and leaving it behind.

Six years after his death, his family will say that he had a good death.

The hospice staff allowed Billy's family to take control of the end of his life. To support them, nurses provided the medication Billy needed to stay comfortable, gave the family privacy, answered their questions, and respected their decisions.

This is an extraordinary case. However, this scenario isn't the norm. In 2002, Last Acts, a national coalition promoting quality end-of-life care, surveyed over 1,000 people in 50 states and graded each state on its provision of end-of-life care. About 60 percent of those surveyed rated care for the dying as fair or lower, and 25 percent rated it as poor. The researchers concluded that Americans "at best have no better than a fair chance of finding good care for their loved ones or themselves when facing a life-threatening illness" (Blacksher, 2002).

Because Billy couldn't take control of the dying process himself, his family did it for him. There was no rush to "911" him to the hospital for futile life-prolonging treatments. There was no conflict between the family and professional caregivers. There was no last-minute expense for the newest technology or medication. No pleas for help.

To explore the concept of a good death, researchers investigated how people want to be cared for at the end of their lives. In one study, chronically-ill patients identified these five goals for quality end-of-life care (Singer, 1999):

1. To avoid inappropriately prolonging dying.
2. To strengthen relationships with loved ones.
3. To relieve the burden on their loved ones.
4. To receive adequate pain and symptom management.
5. To achieve a sense of control.

Billy's family designed the care he received at the end of his life. His family was well-informed about his right to receive individualized and compassionate care and avoid aggressive, expensive, and futile interventions. Supported by his hospice team, they were able to design the care he received at the end of his life. When they buried Billy he was wearing the uniform of his beloved Miami Dolphins.

Statement of the Problem

Poor symptom management at the end of life may impel patient requests to end life via assisted suicide. The desires of terminally-ill patients for hastened death have been associated with depression, hopelessness, pain, and other symptom distress. (Breitbart, et al, 2000). Experience in Oregon, the only state to legalize physician-assisted suicide, is contrary to these findings. Patient requests for lethal medication most frequently involve concerns about loss of autonomy, decreasing ability to participate in activities that make life enjoyable, and loss of control over bodily functions. This finding may reflect sustained efforts in Oregon to improve palliative care. The Oregon Death with Dignity Act also requires that physicians inform patients of alternatives such as hospice, comfort care, and pain control. Patients believed to have a psychological condition that may impair judgment must be referred to a psychiatrist or psychologist for further evaluation (Ganzini et al, 2001).

In other literature, there is a general consensus that medical professionals and nurses should respond to requests for Assisted Death (AD) by examining their own beliefs and values about AD, listening to patient concerns and unmet needs, informing patients about all palliative care options, aggressively managing symptoms, and maintaining a nonjudgmental approach.

Purpose of the Study

The National Institute of Aging reported that 78 million baby boomers (people ages 39 to 57) represent 27.5 percent of the total population. By 2030, the baby boomers will be 66 to 84 and are projected to compose 20 percent of the total population.

Because most of the 2.4 million Americans who die each year are at least 65 and death is an inevitable part of aging, the demand for end-of-life care can be expected to increase as demographics shift (NIH, 2004).

With improved life expectancy, the incidence of chronic disease has increased. Chronic diseases are among the most prevalent, costly, and potentially preventable of all health problems. Approximately 80 percent of people 65 or older have at least one chronic condition, and 50 percent have at least two. In addition, an increasing prevalence of chronic disease is expected to rise with time (NIH, 2004).

Advances in medicine and technology have allowed more and more Americans to live longer with chronic and advanced chronic illness. Patients with chronic disease often suffer from pain and depression, further complicating their management. In addition, variation occurs in the decline in function and health status, as well as progression of the expected course of different chronic diseases. Multiple chronic diseases often coexist, particularly in the elderly, adding to the complexity of disease management (Emanuel et al, 1999).

Despite the best options in medical technology, many patients with advanced, life-limiting illness suffer needlessly in the final stages of their lives. Humane care for those approaching death is a social obligation that is not being met in our communities.

Too often, death is viewed as a medical failure rather than the final chapter to life. As a result, people have come to fear a prolonged and over-treated death, and profound suffering for themselves and their family. Conversation about death is avoided in families and with providers until a crisis occurs, resulting in inadequate advance-care planning and patient preferences that are not honored. Palliative and hospice care is introduced late and is often inadequate.

Importance of the Study

Models of End-Of-Life-Care

Palliative care at the end of life has largely been provided by hospice and financed with the Medicare hospice benefit. Hospice delivers care that neither hastens nor postpones death.

The focus is on maintaining quality of life, including relief from pain and other distressing symptoms, while integrating medical, psychological, and spiritual aspects of care. Support systems are offered for patients to live as actively as possible, and for families during the patient's illness and in bereavement (Last Acts, 2004).

Hospice offers comprehensive care in the last months of life. Services are provided by a multidisciplinary team of doctors, nurses, social workers, pastoral counselors, home health aides, volunteers, and a range of therapists. All services are provided in the home, if at all possible. Otherwise, inpatient care is available in hospice facilities, special hospital units, and nursing homes (Last Acts, 2004).

Despite the fact that hospice is widely available, its services are underused. The average length of treatment in hospice has dropped from 70 days in 1983 to approximately 36 days today. To adequately address physical, emotional, psychosocial, and spiritual needs, experts estimate a dying patient requires at least 60 days of care from hospice (Last Acts, 2004). In 1990, the World Health Organization defined palliative care as "an approach that improves the quality of life of patients and families facing the problem associated with life-threatening illness, through the prevention and relief of suffering by means of early identification and impeccable assessment and treatment of pain and other problems, physical, psychosocial, and spiritual."

On a national level, various models have been tried in an attempt to integrate palliative care into mainstream medicine. Hospital/Hospice collaborations have launched palliative care inpatient teams and units. In this model of palliative care, case managers play a pivotal role in integrating the management of chronic illness by means of disease-modifying treatment with palliative care services and with easing the transition to hospice care.

To better define the cohort of patients who potentially are eligible for hospice and would benefit from a palliative approach, the critical question is, "would it surprise me if this patient died in the next year?"

Scope of the Study

Palliative care (PC) is often recommended by physicians for their patients who are terminally ill. In contrast to hospice care, which precludes the use of any curative treatment at life's end stages, PC seeks primarily to comfort patients and to keep them pain free, yet it does not necessarily preclude medical treatment. It does seek to attend to patients' physical as well as psychological, emotional, spiritual, and existential needs in an attempt to enhance overall quality of life.

Rationale of the Study

The philosophy of palliative care is often used interchangeably with the philosophy of hospice care. Yet, the majority of patients actually die in settings other than hospice. Consequently, there is a need to promote skills in palliative care to healthcare providers in a variety of settings. The influence for the development of this study is the belief that education is the key to the development of new attitudes, knowledge, and skills in palliative care, in order that care for all dying patients should improve.

Overview of Study

End-of-life care is an art. It is a challenging and essential area of medical practice. There is no other specialty with this degree of responsibility. This study explores the fundamentals of palliative care and the support of dying patients. Components of such care include: identifying that death is approaching; discussion with the patient, family, and caregivers; the management of distressing symptoms; and support for all involved.

The study explores the final decline of a progressive illness. Families and patients may perceive signs of imminent death. They may have no specialized knowledge of the dying process but have a unique insight and their impressions often add sensitivity to the identification of end-of-life events.

Sometimes there is a tendency for people to withdraw from a dying person, and professionals are not immune from this. This may be a fear of death or lack of confidence that they will know what to say or do. Very often, little needs to be said or done, but the act of not withdrawing, of continuing to go into the room rather than around it, is valuable in its own right.

One of the hallmarks of palliative care is the involvement in decisions of patients, and where appropriate, families. Examples are decisions such as where the patient may wish to die and the use of possible life-prolonging treatment and possibly futile interventions—for example, antibiotics are withdrawn.

Most patients want doctors to discuss such issues. They may not be able to ask about it openly because of fear and anxiety or may think that they would be wasting the doctor's time. It is not unusual for families to withhold such information from the patients, as they fear its adverse impact. It would be useful again to allay their anxieties and explore reasons for such a request. It should be made clear that if a patient wants to know, it is a doctor's duty to give the patient honest information.

Effective care at the end of life is a multidisciplinary and multiprofessional task. Physicians and nurses are commonly the main professionals, but in some cases there is a need for others' involvement—for example, chaplains, social workers, physical therapists, and possibly the specialist palliative care team. In addition many areas now have community-nursing care or can receive hospice services at home, which undertake care of patients who are dying in the community. Where many professionals are involved good communication and teamwork is essential both between colleagues and with the patient and their family.

Ongoing Evaluation and Symptom Control

Patients' needs at the end of life can be complex. A marked proportion of patients (though not all) will develop new symptoms of worsening or existing symptoms. Patients may not mention these due to exhaustion or the assumption that nothing can be done to help. Full examination may cause discomfort and have little if any role to play in end-of-life care, and procedures such as repeated blood tests are unnecessary and distressing to patients.

Although drugs are a large part of the management of many symptoms at the end of life, it is important to stop some drugs, as it is to start others. Most long-term drugs may be stopped—for example, a dying patient does not need drugs to lower their blood pressure, slow their heart rate, or lower their cholesterol levels.

Palliative care and quality of life issues in patients with terminal illness have become an important area of clinical concern. Perhaps the most clinically-relevant mental health issues in palliative care today are the medical, social, and psychological factors that may contribute to suicide ideation, hastened death, and physician-assisted suicide. Public interest has grown since the media attention devoted to the Florida case of Terry Schiavo. The growing availability of life-extending medical treatment to the terminally ill has opened communication and debate with ethical issues related to end-of-life options.

The Role of the Medical Professional

Social workers, psychologists, and skilled clinicians can work as a team to help the patient and family through the crisis. Palliative care needs to be discussed as the terminally ill fear suffering and dying in pain. Giving pain-relieving medications to patients at regular intervals rather than waiting for their pain to intensify provides better relief for chronic pain. Antidepressant medication can additionally be effective in the relief of pain.

One problem facing the terminally ill is their suicide ideation. It is the role of the physician and other healthcare providers to intervene when their patients begin voicing their suicidal thoughts.

The physician is trained to save lives. However, throughout their training, they are not provided with the tools to assess their patient's values. Those values are significant and what helps to keep the patient alive. However, physicians sometimes create a safe emotional distance from their patient causing the terminally ill to fall deeper into depression. The dying patient, upon noticing that the physician is distant or aloof, feels depersonalized and inhibited from discussing important concerns. This is unfortunate because patients' questions can be an opportunity to provide information that could reassure them about comfort measures that would be implemented as their condition worsens and how their dying could occur with appropriate support.

Reasons for Seeking Hastened Death/PAS

A growing body of literature has emerged indicating the types of physical and psychological concerns that may give rise to a desire for hastened death and requests for assisted suicide. Specifically, the issues that have received the broadest empirical support are pain, depression, social support, and cognitive dysfunction.

If patients received proper counseling and were assured their needs would be met, perhaps they would not choose the option of physician-assisted suicide.

What the terminally ill require is that physicians not neglect them as concerns and fears are communicated. The concerns can include pain and personal image, particularly as they grow weaker and notice dramatic physical changes in themselves, loss of bodily functions, unfinished business, the need to remain in control of their treatment decisions and having access to the truth.

Easing much of a dying patient's pain is medically possible. Their body, mind, and spirit should never be neglected. The neglect and the fear lead to depression. As complete sadness and overwhelming despair engulf the terminally ill, their thinking can become irrational.

The acceptable practice of discussing physician-assisted suicide and following through with completion of the act became the legal option of terminally-ill Oregon residents on October 27, 1997.

The OHD reports that the terminally-ill Oregon residents can obtain a prescription from their physician for lethal medications as long as the patient is:

> An adult (18 years of age or older); A resident of Oregon; Capable (defined as able to make and communicate health care decisions); Diagnosed with a terminal illness that will lead to death within 6 months. Patients who meet these requirements are eligible to request a prescription for lethal medication from a licensed Oregon physician. To receive a prescription for lethal medication, the following steps must be fulfilled: The patient must make two verbal requests to their physician, separated by at least 15 days; the patient must provide a written request to their physician; the prescribing physician and a consulting physician must determine whether the patient is capable.

> If either physician believes the patient's judgment is impaired by a psychiatric or psychological disorder, such as depression, the patient must be referred for counseling; the prescribing physician must inform the patient of feasible alternatives to assisted suicide including comfort care, hospice care, and pain control; the prescribing physician must request, but may not require, the patient to notify their next-of-kin of the prescription request.

As the terminally ill face critical issues, their physician guides them through treatment options. Benefits are provided to the patient respectfully and fairly and, together, a treatment plan is determined. It is the physician's obligation not to harm the patient and this principle of nonmaleficence must remain intact, as the terminally ill struggle with their life options. Such struggles begin at the moment of learning their prognosis to the day of their death. Some terminally-ill patients may undergo treatment and then request PAS. Others may request PAS upon learning of a prognosis of having less than six months to live and not opt for any life-saving measures.

The Role of Family and Cultural Values

The role of the family is an important consideration in end-of-life care. Cultural beliefs, customs and rituals, bring comfort to the entire family. Emotional, physical, and spiritual needs of the dying are met as clergy and family play a critical role in the care. As the condition of the patient deteriorates, the entire family is affected. Physicians should provide families with options that offer information on various aspects of their loved one's health care. Physicians need to respect the family's beliefs, and in so doing, be mindful not to stereotype their patient in any way. Patients rely on family for guidance and the physician may have to work with a member of the family before any decision is made in regard to terminal care.

The physician must listen to both the terminally-ill patient and his family as they communicate their needs. The physician must be willing to communicate all options. It is sometimes left to the family to elect certain procedures for their family member. Therefore, the physician must remain confident that through his communication, everyone's needs are being met and everyone in the family understands what is being done and not done.

The burden of care giving and financial responsibilities cannot be ignored. All issues need to be addressed as the family's burden creates additional suffering for the terminally ill. As patients communicate their needs, they take control of their end-of-life care. It begins with devising a plan of action and having an advance directive. This will enable their wishes to be known.

Treatment Modalities

Non-drug therapies share the common features of increasing patients' sense of participation and control, providing interest and occupation when jobs or hobbies have had to be discontinued, and offering a supportive personal relationship. Usually delivered in regular planned sessions, they can also help in acute situations—for example, deep breathing, relaxation techniques, or massage for acute anxiety or panic attacks. Options to ease suffering in the terminally ill include therapeutic touch, which helps the terminally ill by promoting relationships and pain reduction. Music therapy can also be utilized in end-of-life care. Curtis' study of seventeen terminally-ill patients reported (O'Callaghan, 1996) that the music was effective in reduction of pain, physical discomfort, relaxation, and contentment scores. Other studies have found similar findings when the terminally ill listen to taped music. Lane (as cited in O'Callaghan, 1996) reported that listening to music can benefit patients while they are undergoing painful procedures. Physicians can incorporate massage therapy and the use of touch in their patient's care along with any pain medication. Family members can be educated as to the importance of touch, as they may be hesitant to touch; afraid of causing additional pain to their dying loved one. Depending upon the response of the terminally ill, that touch may be exactly what is needed. Zuberbueler (1996) explains that massage reduces pain and slows the skin breakdown. A blending of certain oils and gentle massage is soothing and healing.

The relationship between suicide ideation in the terminally ill and physical and emotional suffering has been briefly explored. A direct solution to the problem of suicide ideation in the terminally ill is educating physicians about more effective pain management. This education can include incorporating family therapy and cognitive-behavioral methods along with complementary therapies in end-of-life care. The review of the literature revealed that the terminally ill who die by assisted suicide are suffering in what they believe to be a helpless and hopeless situation. Physicians must offer them hope that their pain will not be ignored, their stress and psychological concerns will be treated appropriately, and though they may lose control of bodily functions, they will be cared for in a dignified manner. Suicide does not have to be an option for the terminally ill when effective care is in place.

Societal View

Researchers are exploring society's view of suicide, euthanasia, and physician-assisted suicide (PAS). Participants in the studies are made aware of the differences between euthanasia, suicide, and physician-assisted suicide. PAS is defined as any action designed to terminate the life of a seriously-ill individual who requests such assistance. The physician provides the means in which the patient dies. The physician does not personally intervene and the patient ends his own life. Euthanasia refers to the physician's intervention, whereby an active role is taken in ending the patient's life. The physician eases his patient's suffering and allows for a good death.

There are several types of suicide. "Discussed" assisted suicide is where the physician discusses alternatives and encourages all options. "Accepted" assisted suicide is where little if any discussion of options is discussed. "Encouraged" assisted suicide is where the physician encourages ending one's life and may provide the means to do so. Lastly, "Suicide," where the individual finds the means himself and ends his life with or without the knowledge of others.

In these situations, the patient is clearly saying he or she wants his or her emotional or physical pain alleviated and that he or she cannot live with the pain or the depression that clouds their judgment.

Depression

The findings of the literature review clearly show that there is a need to end suffering, and the means to that end does not have to be suicide.

Assistance can be offered to those who fear death, fear becoming a burden to family, and fear losing their dignity. Research shows that depression stems from physical pain. Pain and suffering affect one's physical function and social interaction. One's coping mechanisms, support system, and physician's powerful influence are important considerations. These attachments can keep one from ending his life when he is overwhelmed with pain.

The emotional and cognitive changes in patients with advanced disease reflect both psychological and biological effects of the medical condition and its treatment. Psychological adjustment reactions after diagnosis or relapse often include fear, sadness, perplexity, and anger. These usually resolve within a few weeks with the help of the patients' own personal resources, family support, and professional care.

Methodology

An extensive literature review demonstrated the enormous amount of research on end-of-life issues and assisted death. In contrast, the research data provided a unique source of analysis and insights into the personal problems encountered in terminal care. The literature review was almost exclusively based on survey research methodology. Little of it gave insight into the day-to-day struggles and personal perspectives of the study participants. The approach utilized an opportunity to make the lived experiences directly available to the researcher. This was accomplished by listening, recording and analyzing the participant's stories about those crises that have resulted in major changes in their thoughts about terminal care. In the case of the participants in this study, these moments forced them to reflect deeply on their personal values, attitudes, and beliefs.

The Approach

This qualitative study aimed to explore symptom management strategies utilized in lieu of providing assisted death to terminally-ill persons. The research question was this: What are the symptom management strategies used to prevent or respond to requests for AD from terminally-ill patients? The study evolved into an analysis of written stories from 12 nurses who agreed to describe their experiences with a request for assisted dying. What had started out as research into palliative care and end-of-life issues became a subset of just two questions about assisted death.

The Data Gathering Method

Following a literature review, conclusions were drawn by what was omitted from previous studies conducted. Essentially, this helped shape the focus and direction of the study. Key included nurse case managers, social workers, and physicians.

The research and interview questions that these individuals would be asked included an overall health needs assessment based on "terminal stage" of their patients. The majority of questionnaires returned were from nursing and case management personnel. This finding was explored and ultimately led to the secondary analysis phase. All respondents felt that nursing relationships were the strongest since they are most directly involved with terminal patients and their care. Additionally, "floor staff" seemed more candid about their experiences while on terminal care units. Physicians were more inclined to refer their patients to hospice and remove themselves from the terminal care of the patient.

Two themes emerged from the participant's stories:

- Alternative strategies for AD
- Prevention of requests for AD

The participants shared many examples of clinical interventions to relieve or prevent suffering including physical, emotional, and spiritual care practices; comfort and medication management; and service as teacher-advocate. Both those who had received requests for AD and those who had not used a variety of similar symptom management approaches to alleviate suffering. The secondary analysis of the stories not previously analyzed were from the perspective of symptom management. The sample for this analysis consisted of 12 stories from nurses and nurse case managers who had: a) received no requests for AD but submitted commentary on symptom management practices and experiences with end-of-life care and; b) nurses who had received and denied requests for AD but countered with symptom management strategies. Hence, none of the sample for the current study stated that they had engaged in AD. The recipients who chose to participate were requested to submit a written response to the following directions:

- Describe a situation in which you received a request from a terminally-ill patient to assist dying. This could be a situation in which you chose to assist or declined to assist. Assistance could assume the form of taking action to end life such as administering a lethal drug dose, advising a patient about specific strategies or available resources for ending life, assisting the patient with an act to end life, or refraining from interventions to prevent or dissuade the patient from taking his or her life.

• Describe your experience, including your thoughts and feelings at the time and in retrospect, as fully as you can.

Validity, Originality and Limitation of Data

Descriptions of symptom management strategies used to address requests for AD were obtained through analysis of written stories submitted by nurses, physicians, and social workers. The analysis addressed the experience of receiving requests for AD.

The researcher, however, also received correspondence from those who denied ever receiving requests for AD. These individuals described symptom management practices that they stated had prevented such requests. Although one group of participants received requests for AD whereas the other did not, both groups shared many examples of using symptom control strategies to care for people within the context of dying. The interventions they used were consistent with current recommendations to implement comfort care strategies in response to requests for AD. The study participants instituted actions according to established standards in response to an ethically-troubling patient request.

Currently, no studies have been done that directly support measurable indicators specific to dignified dying and sensitive to individual patient preferences regarding symptom management and control over the dying process. Terminal care and hospice nurses seem ideally positioned to provide leadership in outcomes research for end-of-life care strategies.

The current study included a subset of respondents who received requests for AD, denied those requests, and countered with symptom management strategies. Did denial of the patient request and implementation of such strategies represent only one of numerous steps the respondents took to explore a patient's request for AD? Is such a refusal consistent with the advocacy role of nursing and the value placed on a patient's right to self-determination?

Summary

The demographic profile shows a predominantly Christian group of women with an average age of 45.5 years (range, 24-67 years). This group had experience, averaging 21.5 years (range, 3-40 years) of nursing practice and 15 years (range, 0.3-30 years) of critical care practice. Most of the nurses were employed full-time in direct care roles. The participants in the study resided in Palm Beach County.

The physicians in the study were predominantly Jewish males with an average age of 46.5 (range, 37-56). They had spent their entire careers in medicine. While for a majority of the women, it was a second career choice.

Data Analysis

As a part of the study 12 informants responded to the survey. These people represented professionals from the Palm Beach County medical community. The respondents were anonymous. The questions presented in this were selected as questions that best represent the observations about the quality of palliative care and terminal illness and what defines a "good death."

The Survey

The following are summaries of the questions and answers from the survey.

Alternative Strategies to Assisted Dying

Palliative care measures and hospice referrals were implemented by the nurses who received and denied requests for AD. Their stories were characterized by alternative strategies to AD, defined as physical, emotional, and spiritual symptom management strategies used in response to patient or family member requests for AD. Pain management was a predominant issue. For example, one nurse stated: "I refused to give extra doses of morphine for that purpose [of ending life] but was readily available to provide medication to control pain, anxiety, or respiratory distress. I did readjust the IV dose as needed, based on clinical judgment, not to hasten the patient's death."

Similarly, a hospice nurse shared an experience reflecting an initial encounter with a patient she was admitting to hospice care. The patient asked, "Can't you do something to end my life now?" She responded that she could not fulfill that request, but said: "My job will be to eliminate as much pain as possible and to keep you comfortable at home. Pain management starts today, and before I leave, you will be more comfortable. Medication will be left to take on an 'as needed' basis to ensure that you are not in any pain or discomfort."

Another care manager shared her personal philosophy of end-of-life care as a response to requests for AD. She stated that she saw her role as that of an educator for families and patients. She then shared an example of how she managed both physical and emotional distress, describing her care of a dying man with AIDS and his family. She described interventions used to help them overcome myths about morphine and addiction, to treat them with positive regard, and to assist the man in regaining a sense of self-esteem:

> His family had convinced him that taking meds for pain would make him an addict. Their family member was terminal. At what point does addiction matter? By the time of his death, everyone felt that the treatment given was the best possible.

> Other nurses spoke of other responses to requests for AD, such as exploring patients' requests, identifying fears, and instituting measures to alleviate those fears. Most respondents described fear of a potentially painful death as the patient's major concern.

The following example epitomizes the stories of those who instituted aggressive symptom management to control physical and emotional symptom distress:

> Annette admitted that it was pain that concerned her the most. We made an informal contract that day that I would work closely with her physician to provide pain and symptom management so that she, hopefully, would not reach the point of needing to take her own life. For the next several months, her family, physician, and I worked diligently in adjusting medications to control her pain, anxiety, and depression.

One participant shared a spiritual care intervention. She described a dying patient that she admitted with uncontrolled pain from advanced metastatic breast cancer. She stated that after a morphine drip had been initiated and the patient's pain had become more controlled, she continued to request to be "let go." "Addressing her fear, which became more obvious as the pain subsided, I asked her if she had a faith. Yes, she believed in Christ and considered herself deeply spiritual. We talked about Christ and her beliefs about death and the afterlife. While some others might have found this inappropriate, in this case it made the patient more comfortable. It gave her something to hold onto. The patient had a deep spiritual conviction that she would be with her Lord. This patient's symptom distress was responded to by addressing the spiritual component." One nurse summarized a philosophy that paralleled the opinions of many nurses who told stories of refusing requests and implementing palliative care:

> Dying is hard work. In my 21 years, I have learned that hard work is needed to fight cancer. Work to treat and deal with side effects helps people get to a cure or to have time to live and have closure. Assisted suicide is against my beliefs, and I give patients and their families caring, help, assistance, explanations, and presence. Often, just being there is enough. Feeling that they are burdens causes the need to have it be over, to die.

Preventing Requests for Assisted Dying

Stories were also submitted associated with managing symptoms that prevent patient requests for AD. One case manager stated, "the first great lesson I learned from team conferences and patient rounds were that you couldn't catch up to pain. You need to start pain management in anticipation of future pain. I have been able to control pain and symptom management in my patients. Therefore, I have not been faced with this situation."

The theme of preventing requests for AD was defined as perceived prevention of requests for AD via management of comfort care practices and acting as teacher/advocate. One social worker described this as follows: "In all of my years in end-of-life care and now practicing as a palliative care practitioner, I have never had one of my patients request to die. I believe that because I have worked with very strong interdisciplinary teams and have learned to treat depression early on and know how to properly manage pain and symptoms, my patients die 'good' deaths."

Other respondents included comments about managing medications at the end of life: "Although I have never been formally asked by a patient to assist with termination of their lives as in advising strategies, I have given full doses of meds as opposed to partial orders actually written."

Another nurse offered her perspective:

> Chasing symptoms with multiple meds is something I frequently see in many hospice programs. If I come to a place in my patient's care that dictates sedation for unrelieved symptoms after numerous trials of meds, I will offer sedation on an "as needed" basis for breakthrough pain. I guess this can be seen as terminal sedation.

Terminal sedation is the use of sedatives to relieve extreme, intractable physical distress in the final days of life. Because the intent is to relieve suffering by rendering the patient unconscious and not to hasten death, the practice is ethically and legally supported as a symptom management strategy.

Other comments about end-of-life care focused on the importance of patient counseling, teaching, and advocacy: "As a chemotherapy treatment nurse, I have often wanted to discuss Hospice with various patients who I believed would benefit from the hospice support team, along with their families and loved ones. I believe in quality versus quantity, and the patients often need to be aware of other options, especially when so many treatments have failed and they are feeling miserable on a regular basis. I believe nurses in my field need to be advocates. Similarly, I have helped rearrange pain management plans, defined "terminal" to patients, and discussed the merits of hospice on numerous occasions. I have discussed at length the quality of eating, sleeping, moving, pursuing pleasurable goals, general 'living' to many patients and their families in order for them to make an informed choice between life and death. I have had one chemo patient state to me 'this isn't living, it's existing.' If that is the case, other options should be given."

In summary, both the respondents who received requests for AD and those who did not share many examples of clinical interventions and other features used to control suffering at the end of life. The first theme, alternatives to AD, represented symptom management strategies that nurses implemented in response to a patient or family request for AD. The second theme, preventing requests for AD, included symptom management strategies that practitioners believed prevented patients from seeking AD.

Assessing and Managing Depression in the Terminally-Ill Patient

Respondents in the survey strongly reacted to questions of mental health and depression. Three case studies were reviewed to illustrate the assessment and management of normal or appropriate grieving, the diagnosis and treatment of depression, and the assessment and management of suicidal ideation in terminally-ill patients. Respondents felt skillful management of depression relieves suffering and is a core element of the provision of comprehensive end-of-life care. Although treatment of pain and other symptoms at the end of life has improved, they felt that depression and other psychological symptoms and disorders remain troublesome for terminally-ill patients. Many of these conditions can be easily controlled with psychosocial treatments. Respondents stated that physicians who care for dying patients should be competent in this critical area of clinical practice. The result was an overwhelming response of how mental health issues integrate with palliative care.

Psychological distress often causes suffering in terminally-ill patients and their families and poses challenges in diagnosis and treatment. Increased attention to diagnosis and treatment of depression can improve the coping mechanisms of patients and thus their families.

Three cases were utilized to illustrate assessment and management of normal distress and grieving, clinical depression, and the wish to hasten death in the presence of psychological distress.

Case One: Sadness, Grief, or Depression?

Mr. Roberts, a 53-year-old man with late-stage Parkinsons, is cared for at home by his wife and the local hospice program. He receives long-term oxygen therapy, is bedridden, and has been hospitalized in the past year for respiratory failure that required ventilatory support and secondary infections. Mr. Roberts is concerned about becoming a burden to his wife. Their income is barely enough to meet their needs. Recently, the hospice nurse has expressed concern about Mr. Roberts's mental state because he has been asking repeatedly why he has to wait around to die. When directly questioned, he states that he has no intention of ending his life but that he is distressed by his helplessness and dependence. He spends his time watching television and trying to complete simple projects.

The physician who hears this report must assess the severity of Mr. Roberts's distress. Is he depressed, or is he experiencing normal grieving that is part of the dying process? In addition, the physician must confront the challenge of bearing with the patient's distress and remaining an ally while the patient walks this difficult path.

The physician makes a house call to assess Mr. Roberts's condition. Throughout the visit, Mr. Roberts makes jokes about his condition and repeatedly refers to his death in a joking manner. Through questioning, the physician learns that Mr. Roberts is not sleeping well because he is short of breath and anxious about not waking up, that his appetite is poor, and that he has little energy. He reports that he does not want to see anyone except his family and that he lacks the concentration and focus to read. When asked whether he is depressed, Mr. Roberts replies, "Angry, yes. Worried about my wife, yes. But depression? No."

He remarks on how much he enjoys his projects and how he worries that he will not have time to complete them. Mr. Roberts reports that he is realistic about his prognosis, hopes for a few more months, is trying to do as much as possible for himself, and is not suicidal. He says that joking has always been his way of coping with difficult situations.

Respondents:

Mr. Roberts's case presents many of the common challenges in diagnosing depression. He has several of the symptoms of depression (difficulty sleeping, poor appetite, loss of energy, and diminished concentration). However, these symptoms may be caused or exacerbated by underlying disease. Mr. Roberts is also grieving as he anticipates his death. His withdrawal from people other than his family is part of the normal grieving process, particularly because he continues to enjoy his family. Like other terminally-ill patients, he expresses ambivalence about the prospect of death, simultaneously accepting and denying it.

The single question "Are you depressed?" provides a sensitive and specific assessment of depression in terminally-ill patients. A patient who responds affirmatively to such an inquiry is likely to receive a diagnosis of depression after a comprehensive diagnostic interview. The clinician can use this question as a screening tool; for example, Mr. Roberts's negative response is important evidence against a diagnosis of depression.

Patients with depression often exhibit feelings of boredom, hopelessness, aversion, and lack of interest in their caregivers. Mr. Roberts's physician notes that he enjoys his patient's sense of humor and is amused by his delight in shocking the hospice nurse with his jokes (further evidence that Mr. Roberts is not depressed).

Mr. Roberts's distress is focused on real issues related to his illness—the burden of care on his family, uncertainty, and distress about loss of control. He retains the capacity to laugh, and to enjoy his family. Therefore, the physician concludes that Mr. Roberts is not depressed and that his distress seems to fall within the rubric of what the DSM-IV calls "adjustment disorders" (DSM, 1994). The physician suggests that the hospice nurse continue to monitor Mr. Roberts's mood and recommends a trial of an antidepressant only if he demonstrates new depressive symptoms.

Because no "bright line" separates depression from grief or adjustment reactions, the physician must assess whether the patient's symptoms have reached the threshold for treatment. Psychological distress requires treatment even when it does not constitute a psychiatric diagnosis.

Mr. Roberts dies peacefully at home 3 months later.

Case Two: The Assessment and Management of Depression

Ms. Smith is a 44-year-old woman with breast cancer with bone and lung metastases who is receiving palliative chemotherapy. She is Roman Catholic and lives with her husband and two young children. In the past 6 months, she has fractured two vertebrae and has been hospitalized for shortness of breath and fluid in her lungs. She and her family have always wanted aggressive treatment, primarily so that she could continue to be a mother to her children. Recently, however, she said that she is in too much pain to be of help to anyone and that she does not want further treatment. Her pain is poorly controlled with naproxen and morphine; on a 10-point scale, her current pain level is at best a 3 and at worst a 10. She notes that pain often interferes with her sleep and that she cannot sleep past 4:00 a.m. Her appetite is poor, and she has lost interest in her hobbies.

Because of the change in her status, the physician carries out a depression assessment. When asked about her future, Ms. Smith responds: "My future is over. There is nothing ahead for me. I worry about how much suffering is ahead, about my children, and about how my husband will manage. If it weren't for my religion, I don't know what I would do. I used to feel proud of being a good mother and wife. But I've lost that. I have been doing this for three years. I'm done." When asked whether she thinks she is depressed, Ms. Smith says that she is nervous and sad and that she feels that anyone would be depressed in her circumstances.

Respondents:

> Several factors indicate that Ms. Smith is depressed. Physicians caring for terminally-ill patients should consider the diagnosis of depression when a patient unexpectedly elects to discontinue treatment, is experiencing unrelieved pain, or demonstrates any of the psychological symptoms of depression. A clinician can fully evaluate depressive symptoms in this clinical context by asking such questions as "How do you see your future?", "What do you imagine is ahead for you with this illness?", "What aspects of your life do you feel most proud of? Most troubled by?" and "Are you depressed?" Ms. Smith's responses to her physician's questions suggest that she is feeling hopeless and depressed. She is unable to imagine anything positive in her future, feels unable to contribute, and believes that her presence is only a burden to others. Although her religious beliefs make suicide unlikely, she clearly has some wish to end her life.

Suicide ideation and feelings of hopelessness, helplessness, worthlessness, and guilt—all of which are present in Ms. Smith—are among the best indicators of depression in terminally-ill patients. Anxiety usually coexists with depression, and some patients experience an anxious depression.

How Should Depression Be Treated in a Terminally-Ill Patient?

The first step in assessing and treating depression is controlling pain. Uncontrolled pain is a major risk factor for depression and suicide among patients with cancer.

The doses of Ms. Smith's analgesic agents were increased, and her pain control improved. Although her mood brightened slightly, she continued to express hopelessness about the future and her other mood symptoms did not improve.

Respondents:

> Major depression is a treatable condition, even in persons who are terminally ill. Because treatments are usually relatively benign, clinicians should have a low threshold for initiating treatment. Trials of individual interventions demonstrate the effectiveness of psychotherapeutic interventions in relieving distress, improving quality of life, and even prolonging life. We see the effectiveness of psychotropic interventions in relieving depressive symptoms and alleviating psychological distress. An approach that combines supportive psychotherapy, patient and family education, and antidepressants appears to be effective.

When developing a treatment strategy, the clinician must actively question the patient to elicit concerns about death and the dying process, fears about the effect of illness on family members, and past experiences with loss. By addressing these concerns, the physician can help the patient connect with past strengths and assets and spiritual and religious resources, thereby enhancing self-esteem and coping ability. Sometimes, supportive therapy alone is enough to treat depression. Supportive therapy can be provided by a psychiatrist, psychologist, social worker, pastoral counselor, hospice nurse, or primary care physician, depending on time, interest, training, and the severity of the patient's condition. Terminally-ill patients benefit from an approach that combines emotional support, flexibility, appreciation of the patient's strengths, and elements of life review.

This helps the patient develop a sense of closure and completion. Patients with severe depressive symptoms may be too immobilized, hopeless, and dysphoric to effectively engage in psychotherapy; they may first need to receive appropriate antidepressant medication.

Psychostimulants and antidepressants are the mainstay of treatment for depressed, terminally-ill patients.

They are particularly useful for patients who are seriously ill and unable to engage in psychotherapy. Although Ms. Smith is reluctant to start medication she agrees to start a psychostimulant. In two days, her family notes that she has more energy, is sleeping better, and reports less pain. The dose is then increased. Several days later, Ms. Smith reports that she is feeling less downhearted and that although she does not want any more aggressive treatment, she is looking forward to the holidays. In 10 days, Ms. Smith's family feels that she has fully recovered from her depression. She enters a hospice program, and her medication is maintained without recurrence of depressive symptoms.

After her death, Ms. Smith's family expresses their gratitude that "she remained herself until the very end."

In understanding and treating depression, the clinician must recognize that meanings and expression of depressive symptoms vary across cultures. Some patients who strongly believe in an afterlife may struggle to view death as an opportunity to be closer to God, and others may fear hell and damnation. These beliefs influence the patient's response to the crisis of terminal illness.

Case Three: Assessment and Management of Suicidal Ideation in Terminally-Ill Patients

Billy is a 36-year-old man with AIDS who recently stopped receiving antiretroviral treatment because of side effects. He lives with his family and has recently stopped working because he was too ill but has remained active in his church and community. Billy has been open with his family and physician about his intention to end his life if his suffering becomes unbearable.

Over the past several months, Billy has become cognitively impaired because of AIDs-related dementia and is wheelchair-bound because of peripheral neuropathy. He has lost 35 pounds. Nonetheless, he has continued to be active. One day, he comes to his regularly scheduled visit to say good-bye and to thank his physician for the care that he has received. He says that he plans to end his life. Although Billy has considered suicide as a theoretical option, he now seems to have an immediate plan.

Respondents:

When assessing a patient's risk for suicide, the physician must keep in mind that rates of suicide are higher in patients with medical illness than in healthy persons. Additional risk factors for suicide in terminally-ill patients include advanced age, male sex, a diagnosis of cancer or AIDS, depression, hopelessness, delirium, exhaustion, pain, preexisting psychopathology, and a personal or family history of suicide.

Billy, like many patients with life-threatening illnesses, has had frequent suicidal thoughts. In our unit such thoughts occur in many terminally-ill patients with AIDS, and seem to be associated with feelings of loss of control and anxiety about the future. However, a few of our terminal patients expressed a sustained wish for death to come quickly. These patients received a diagnosis of depression and were found to have increased levels of pain and limited social support. Even patients who present the desire for suicide as a "rational" choice should receive a comprehensive assessment.

When assessing the likelihood of depression in a terminally-ill patient, the physician must both remain involved and rely on the expertise of other members of an interdisciplinary team. Several circumstances should prompt a referral to a psychiatrist. A psychiatrist can provide an in-depth assessment of the patient's judgment, decision-making capacity, and mood. A social worker can provide critical information about the patient's social network and coping.

The current standard of practice on our unit suggests that patients should be referred to a psychiatrist for assessment and treatment because of their high risk for suicide. Hallucinations or delusions in depressed patients are viewed as indicators of high risk for suicide. Organic mental disorders are also risk factors, especially among patients with AIDS.

The physician explores Billy's decision to end his life now and asks the social worker and chaplain for their input. Although Billy is initially angry that the physician questions his intention to kill himself, his anger dissipates and he begins to cry when his physician says, "We've been through this disease together. I am not going to abandon you now. We both know that your time is short, but I want to help you have the best possible death you can have." Billy states that he is tired and he is afraid of letting people down by giving up. He says, "I never thought I would say this, but I want to go."

With Billy's agreement, the physician and social worker arrange a family meeting where these concerns are shared. His family explains that they have recognized how exhausted he has become but have been afraid to discuss this with him because they do not want to demoralize him. After the meeting, Billy says that he feels relieved that he does not have to work so hard to keep up appearances. He gives up his community activities, spending his days in bed, and dies 1 month later. His family states that he has had a "good death."

Discussion

Three cases were reviewed to illustrate the assessment and management of normal or appropriate grieving, the diagnosis and treatment of depression, and the assessment and management of suicidal ideation in terminally-ill patients. Skillful management of depression relieves suffering and is a core element of the provision of comprehensive end-of-life care. Although treatment of pain and other symptoms at the end of life has improved, depression and other psychological symptoms and disorders remain troublesome for terminally-ill patients. Many of these conditions can be easily controlled with state-of-the-art psychosocial treatments. Physicians who care for dying patients must be competent in this area of clinical practice.

Discussion and Implications

Despite the use of currently recommended strategies for end-of-life care, some of the stories reflected encounters with patients whose pain was poorly managed. For example, the hospice nurse's statement that "pain management starts today" raises several questions. Why did it take a patient's request for "something that will end my life" to initiate a program of pain management? Where was the medical team who had been providing care for this patient before the hospice nurse who was confronted with this desperate request? Expert pain management and other symptom control must remain an essential component in the advocacy role in patient care.

Many felt that their basic nursing and medical education provided inadequate preparation for end-of-life care. In the current study nurses' comments suggested confusion about the intent of palliative care interventions, and that they may have misinterpreted such actions as hastening death.

Currently, there is little research to support measurable indicators specific to dignified dying and sensitive to individual patient preferences regarding symptom management and control over the dying process.

The current study included a subset of respondents who received requests for AD, denied those requests, and countered with symptom management strategies. Did denial of the patient request and implementation of such strategies represent only one of numerous steps the respondents took to explore a patient's request for AD? Did the denial represent a decision to uphold professional or even personal values regarding nursing's role in the care of patients who seek to control timing or circumstances associated with dying? Although refusal to participate in ending a patient's life is consistent with ethical code is such a refusal consistent with the advocacy role and the value placed on a patient's right to self-determination?

Although some nurses in this study had not experienced requests for AD, they took the time to write out and send lengthy explanations of their roles and experience with end-of-life care. These nurses also may have been more skilled at palliative care and thus did not receive requests for AD because they managed patient and family needs at the end of life better than the other study participants.

Conclusion

This report explored beliefs and experiences with the use of symptom management strategies to prevent or respond to requests for AD at the end of life. The findings suggest perceived success in improving care through symptom management strategies.

Studies have generally supported the hypothesis that severe pain can result in a heightened desire for death. Effective communication among family, patient, and physician is essential to reducing suicide ideation. A study by Ferrell et al found that in addition to patient related factors, family perceptions of pain, caregiver burden, caregiver moods, and differences in caregiver experiences are all factors, which may impact upon pain management and terminal care.

The patient's family includes people of various ages. Each has his or her own attitude about death and dying and brings this belief system to terminal care. The role of the care management team becomes one of treating illness and the pain associated with that illness, and in providing information and support to the patient's family. The attitudes of the family members play an important role in suicide ideation, palliative and terminal care.

Families play an important role in providing terminal care for their loved one. As caregivers they have a unique opportunity to express their thoughts and feelings as part of the grieving process and in discussing imminent death with their family member. Included in their provision of terminal care is to reassure the patient that they will not be abandoned and to allow the patient the opportunity to express themselves as well. All large issues must be dealt with as part of the closure process, such as the parent who has never told her child she was proud of it, or the sibling rivalry that must finally be put to rest.

The discussion of death and the provision of terminal care can be graceful and retrospective, the results of this journey can be surprising. The basis of all techniques are open discussion, the act of expressing personal feelings, and listening while others express them are effective in the provision of terminal care.

References

Breitbart W. Cancer pain and suicide. In: Foley K., Bonica J. J., Ventafridda V., eds. *Advances in Pain Research and Therapy*, Vol 16. New York: Raven Press, 1990: 399-412.

Brown, J. H., Henteleff P., Barakat S. et al. Is it normal for terminally ill patients to desire death? *Am J Psychiatry*. 1986: 143: 208-211.

Chochinov, H. M., Wilson, K. G., Enns, M. et al. Prevalence of depression in the terminally ill: effects of diagnostic criteria and symptom threshold judgments. *Am J Psychiatry*. 1994: 151: 537-540.

Chochinov H. M., Wilson K. G., Enns M. et al. Desire for death in the terminally ill. *Am J Psychiatry*. 1995: 152: 1185-1191.

Chochinov H. M., Wilson K. G., Enns, M., Lander, S.: Are you depressed? Screening for depression in the terminally ill. *Am J Psychiatry*. 1997: 154: 674-676.

Chronic pain: Hope through research [Website]. 1997. National Institute of Neurological Disorders and Stroke, National Institute of Health. Retrieved from the World Wide Web: *http://www.thebody.com/nih/pain/toc.html*.

Cleeland, C. S. The impact of pain on patients with cancer. *Cancer*. 1984: 54: 263-267.

Ellis, V., Hill, J., & Campbell, H. (1995). Hospice techniques: Strengthening the family unit through the healing power of massage. *The American Journal of Hospice & Palliative Care*. July/August. 19-21.

Emanuel, E. J. (1999). What is the great benefit of legalizing euthanasia or physician-assisted suicide? *An International Journal of Social, Political and Legal Philosophy* 109. 629-642.

Emanuel, E. J., Fairclough, D. L., Daniels, E. R. et al. Euthanasia and physician-assisted suicide: attitudes and experiences of oncology patients, oncologists, and the public. *Lancet*. 1996: 347: 1805-1810.

Emanuel, E. J., Fairclough, D. L., Slutsman, J., Alpert, H., Baldwin, D., Emanuel, L. L.: Assistance from family members, friends, paid care givers, and volunteers in the care of terminally ill patients. *N Engl J Med.* 1999, 341:956-63.

Farberow, N. L., Ganzler S., Cuter F., and Reynolds D. An eight year survey of hospital suicides. *Suicide Life Threat Behav.* 1971: 1: 198-201.

Ganzini, L., Fenn, D. S., Lee, M. L. et al. Attitudes of Oregon psychiatrists toward physician-assisted suicide. *Am J Psychiatry.* 1996: 153: 1469-1475.

Gostin, L. O. (1997). Health law and ethics: Deciding life and death in the courtroom. *The Journal of the American Medical Association.* 278. 1523-1528.

Health Division Center for Disease Prevention and Epidemiology. Portland, Oregon. Retrieved March 20, 1999 from the World Wide Web: *http://www.ohd.hr.state.or.us/cdpe/chs/pas/ar-index.htm.* Health Division Center for Disease Prevention and Epidemiology. Portland, Oregon. Retrieved March 20, 1999 from the World Wide Web: *http://www.ohd.hr.state.or.us/cdpe/chs/pas/ar-index.htm.*

Henderson, Charles W. (July 21, 1997). Experimental AIDS Drug Now Available to Some Children. *AIDS Weekly Plus,* p. 24.

Hinton J. Psychiatric consultation in fatal illness. *Proc R Soc Med.* 1972: 65: 1035-1038.

Holland J. C. Psychological aspects of cancer. In: Holland J. F., Frei E., eds. *Cancer Medicine,* 2nd ed. Philadelphia: Lea and Febiger, 1982.[j147] 29a.

Humphry, D. *Final Exit: the Practicalities of Self-Deliverance and Assisted Suicide for the Dying.* Eugene, OR: The Hemlock Society and Secaucus, NJ: Carol Publishing, 1991. [J47] 30.

Ingham, J. & Portenoy R. K.: The measurement of pain and other symptoms. In: *Oxford Textbook of Palliative Medicine.* 2nd Edition (Edited by: Doyle D., Hanks G. W. C., MacDonald N., eds). Oxford, England: Oxford University Press 1998, 203-219.

Levy R. M., Bredesen D. E., & Rosenblum M.L.. Neurological manifestations of the AIDS experience at UCSF and review of the literature. *J Neurosurg* 1985: 62: 475-495.

Lichter, I. (1991). Some psychological causes of distress in the terminally ill. *Palliative Medicine,* 5. 138-146.

O'Callaghan, C.C. (1996). Complementary therapies in terminal care: Pain, music creativity and music therapy in palliative care. *The American Journal of Hospice & Palliative Care,* March/April: 43-49.

Orbach, I., Palgi, Y., Stein, D., Har-Evan, D., Lotem-Peleg, M., Asherov J., & Elizur, A. (1996) *Death Studies,* 20: 327-340.

Oregon State Supreme Court. ORS127-885, 4.01.

Orr, D., O'Dowd, M. A., McKegney F. P., & Natali C. A comparison of self reported suicidal behaviors in different stages of HIV infection (abstract). IV International AIDS Conference, June 21-24, 1990, San Francisco, CA.

Prawl, J. (1998). Health care providers' professional and personal attitudes: Effects on treatment of terminally ill patients. *The Thanatology Newsletter,* 5, 7-16.

Robert Wood Johnson Foundation. (1997). Last Acts Series. Sponsored by the Boston Globe in association with PBS and the Robert Wood Johnson Foundation in New Jersey. At: *www.pbs.org.*

Salzman, C.: Practical considerations for the treatment of depression in elderly and very elderly long-term care patients. *J Clin Psychiatry,* 1999, 60(Suppl 20): 30-3.

Siegel, K. & Tucker, P. Rational Suicide and the terminally ill cancer patient. *Omega,* 1984: 15: 263-269.

Storey, P. & Knight C. F. UNIPAC 2: Alleviating psychological and spiritual pain in the terminally ill. Reston, VA: American Academy of Hospice and Palliative Medicine. 1997, 23-28.

Storey P. & Knight C. F. UNIPAC Four: Management of selected nonpain symptoms in the terminally ill. *Hospice/Palliative Care Training for Physicians: A Self-study Program.* Gainesville, FL: American Academy of Hospice and Palliative Medicine. 1996.

Storey P. & Knight C. F. UNIPAC 3: Assessment and treatment of pain in the terminally ill. Reston, VA: American Academy of Hospice and Palliative Medicine. 1997: 7-18.

Van Der Maas, P. J., an Delden, J. J., Pijnenborg, L. et al. Euthanasia and other medical decisions concerning the end of life. *Lancet.* 1991: 338: 669-674.

Zuberbueler, E. (1996). Complementary therapies in terminal care, Massage therapy: An added dimension in terminal care. *The American Journal of Hospice & Palliative Care*, March/April. 50.

Zucker, A. (1995). The right to die. *Death Studies*, 19: 293-298. The ABC of palliative care is edited by Marie Fallon, Marie Curie senior lecturer in palliative medicine, Beatson Oncology Centre, Western Infirmary, Glasgow, and Bill O'Neill, science and research adviser, British Medical Association, BMA House, London.

Authors' Affilations

Joan D. Atwood, Ph.D., Editor, is the director and founder of Marriage and Family Therapy of New York, Rockville Centre, NY, a counseling center devoted to empowerment and wellness.

Mary E. Canzoneri, M.A., MFT, is a marriage and family therapist at Marriage and Family Therapists of New York, Rockville Centre, NY.

Laura Jean Dreher, M.A., MFT, is a marriage and family therapist at Marriage and Family Therapists of New York, Rockville Centre, NY.

Sandra Farganis, Ph.D., is director of the Wolfson Center for National Affairs, The New School in New York where she also teaches classes in the social sciences.

Concetta Gallo, Ph.D., editor, is a licensed marriage and family therapist.

Jayne Gassman, Ph.D., CMC, is the director of Surrogate Plus, a service dedicated to the care of the adult, and elderly population of Palm Beach County, Florida.

Corinne Kyriacou, Ph.D., Department of Health and Family Studies, Hofstra University.

E. Doyle McCarthy, Ph.D., Department of Sociology, Fordham University.

Anthony R. Quintiliani, Ph.D., LADC, chief psychologist, The Howard Center, ABHS, Burlington, Vermont and Adjunct Graduate Clinical Faculty at The University of Vermont and Southern New Hampshire University-VT Center.

Estelle Weinstein, Ph.D. is a professor of health administration, Department of Health and Family Studies, Hofstra Univeristy.

Daniel W. Wong, Ph.D., is the head of the department and a professor in the Department of Counseling and Educational Psychology, College of Education at Mississippi State University.

Lucy Wong Hernandez, M.S., is an instructor in the Department of Counseling and Educational Psychology, College of Education at Mississippi State University.

Index

Acquired Immune Deficiency Syndrome
(AIDS), 35, 62, 179, 193, 199-201
American Counseling Association
(ACA), 58
American family, 64, 71-72, 79-96
Americans with Disabilities Act (ADA),
62-63
American Psychological Association
(APA), 58-59
assisted death, 181, 189, 190-195, 202

baby boom, 84-86
baby boomers, 93-94, 101
Best, Joel, 168
brutta cosa, 20-25

cancer, 2, 27, 35-37, 47, 62, 100, 193,
197-200
caregiving,
and the elderly, 51-52
balance of power, 33, 104-105, 127
challenges, 62, 202-203
children as caregivers, 52-53
common interventions, 163-166
consequences, 161-163
culturally-based, 65
disengagement, 44, 197
family loyalty, 4, 18-20, 45
family roles, 50
financial strain, 159-160
issues, 53-54
professional caregiving, 180
social construction, 166-172
stress, 173-174
temporary, 49
case studies,
coping with difficult situations, 196-
197
family therapy for adult children
caregivers, 167-168

management of depression, 197-198
narrative family therapy, 12-25
suicide ideations, 199-200
Centers for Disease Control and Prevention (CDC), 63
children,
chronically-ill, 3-6, 35, 47-49
with a chronically-ill parent, 12-25,
52, 110-115
Christensen, Harold, 92
chronic anxiety, 146, 151
chronic illness,
and the elderly, 51, 159-161
biological factors, 30-31
bio-psycho-social perspectives and
approach, 29-30, 54, 68
caregiving, 161-168
complexities, 134-136
couples, 99-100, 121-122
cultural perspectives, 63-65, 76-77
defining, 27, 62, 146
effect on individuals, 3, 28-29, 31-32,
39-40, 65-66, 120-121, 130-131,
134, 139-141
end of life care, 180-182
etiquette, 124-127
impact on families, 1, 8, 15, 24-25,
42-44, 46-47, 54, 67-69, 106-107,
123-124, 129, 132
impact on religious views, 66
impact on young children, 6, 14-17,
20, 35, 47-49, 57-59
memories, 5-6, 112-114, 158
narrative considerations, 138
recommendations for family therapists and caregivers, 69-70
research on treatment, 28
rewards and attention, 3-4
social construction, 32-33, 58, 137-
138, 170-171